THE JAPANESE SKINCARE REVOLUTION

THE JAPANESE SKINCARE REVOLUTION

How to Have the Most Beautiful Skin of Your Life—At Any Age

Chizu Saeki

TRANSLATED BY **Kay Yokota**

PHOTOGRAPHS BY **Hirokazu Takayama**

KODANSHA INTERNATIONAL
Tokyo · New York · London

The publisher gratefully acknowledges the editorial assistance of Mariko Mizui and Kit Pancoast Nagamura, and the cooperation of Agape Inc., the model Mihoko, and the hair & makeup artist Satomi Akizuki.

Distributed in the United States by Kodansha America, LLC, and in the United Kingdom and continental Europe by Kodansha Europe Ltd.

Published by Kodansha International Ltd., 17–14 Otowa 1-chome, Bunkyo-ku, Tokyo 112–8652.

Originally published in Japanese in 2004, in a slightly different form, by Kodansha Ltd. under the title *Bihada Kakumei*.

English publication rights arranged with Kodansha Ltd.

Library of Congress Cataloging-in-Publication Data

Saeki, Chizu.
  [Bihada Kakumei. English]
  The Japanese skincare revolution : how to have the most beautiful skin of your life at any age / Chizu Saeki ; translated by Kay Yokota ; photographs by Hirokazu Takayama. — 1st ed.
      p. cm.
  ISBN 978-4-7700-3083-2
  1. Beauty, Personal. 2. Face—Care and hygiene. 3. Skin—Care and hygiene. I. Title.
  RA778.S18413 2008
  646.7'26—dc22
                        2008035906

www.kodansha-intl.com

CONTENTS

PREFACE

I was 60 years old when I first put my ideas about skincare into a book. I wrote the book because I wanted to share with all women the policies and techniques that I had developed over my 45-year career as a beautician. My message is simple: anyone who desires to be beautiful can be beautiful, and the power to do that is in your own hands.

A major principle of the Saeki method is to get to know your skin and care for it yourself according to its condition. To do this, you make full use of your hands. Your hands are the ultimate tools—they can gauge your skin's condition like a sensor and smooth out wrinkles like an iron. They can also warm and soothe tensed-up skin, making it more receptive to skincare ingredients.

The effectiveness of any skincare product depends greatly on its use. It's how you use your cosmetics, not what you use, that will transform your skin. Whether you only draw 25 dollars' worth out of a 50-dollar product or 100 dollars' worth is up to you.

After earning a professional license at a beauty school, I worked for some time at a beauty salon in the Ginza district of Tokyo before joining the French cosmetics producer Guerlain as a supervisor of human resources. Guerlain takes an analytical approach to skincare, focusing on the skin's physiology. It offers eight different kinds of cleansing products alone, for instance, and provides counseling to determine which product best serves each client's skin condition or purpose.

Eventually, my husband's work took us to San Francisco, from where I regularly reported to Japan about the U.S. cosmetics market. Americans have great marketing skills, and I was impressed by sales strategies that played on the psychology of consumers. There was one brand, for instance, that had designed all-white cosmetics counters reminiscent of clinics. I discovered that different countries have different ideas of skincare. American skincare primarily consists of "waking up" the skin, such as by stimulating it with patting or by massaging the face with upward motions. By contrast, the French prefer soothing the skin—wiping away makeup and dirt and conditioning the skin—from a more medical standpoint. Over the course of my career, I obtained the knowledge needed to compare the different methods and choose what is best for each skin type.

At the age of 45, I took up the position of international training manager at Parfums Christian Dior and became responsible for training over 600 cosmetic consultants. Christian Dior is one of the world's top couture brands. But it would be pointless to sell its cosmetics just for the brand they bear. So I set out to train professionals capable of providing first-rate counseling services—with whose help clients can look into the mirror with a hopeful feeling and think, "Yes, I can become more beautiful!" And to that end, I developed a sales manual from scratch. Moreover, when Christian Dior opened its Japanese flagship salon in Tokyo's Imperial Hotel, I had the pleasure of treating clients firsthand as an esthetician. My techniques won the confidence of many clients, and the salon became known for having a waiting list of over 100 people.

As all this illustrates, my skincare method is based on my knowledge of cosmetic products from across the world and my years of experience directly caring for clients' skin.

Having looked at the skin of a great many women over the years, I've gained the ability to find out a lot just by taking a quick glance at someone's skin. At times, I've surprised people by correctly pointing out the particular product and brand they use. Though I may sound to them like a fortune-teller, there actually are certain characteristics that tend to emerge when certain types of products are used. For instance, the Japanese, whose land is blessed with plenty of clean water, love to wash their faces. It's not unusual for a Japanese woman to use a highly detergent oil cleanser, on top of which she'll wash her face again with soap to get rid of the oiliness remaining on her skin. She further burdens the skin, already made vulnerable from too much cleansing, by coating it with expensive cream to alleviate the dryness. The more a person is dedicated to skincare, the more she is prone to jump on new and potent products, thereby further ruining her skin.

Whether cleansers or pricey creams, cosmetics are made for the purpose of beautifying the skin. But if used incorrectly, they can also do harm. In the final analysis, it is you and only you who can care for and protect your skin. I would like to bestow on everyone the knowledge and techniques to do this successfully.

I've adored beautiful things from a very young age, and I was particularly fascinated by Hollywood movies. In fact, my interest in cosmetics stems from my infatuation with the actress Audrey Hepburn and my desire to be like her. The glittery, glorious world on the silver screen, exemplified in makeup by artists such as Max Factor and Helena Rubenstein, has given me dreams.

It's only when you use cosmetics correctly that you can draw out their full potential and obtain beautiful skin. How wonderful if women the world over were able to achieve this with my techniques! That is my way of repaying the world with all my heart for the dreams I was given as a young girl.

Chizu Saeki
May 2008

The Tenets of Saeki-style Skincare

Don't worry about every spot and wrinkle. It's the overall demeanor and luster of your face that determine the impression you give.

Get the most out of your skincare products

My approach to skincare always meets with surprise. "Why didn't I ever think of that before?" people say when I demonstrate my methods, or "What a great idea!" But all I'm doing, really, is adding a few extra touches to perfectly commonplace techniques.

There's nothing special about the products I use, just how I use them. For example, instead of applying lotion directly to my skin, I squirt a few drops onto a wet cotton square and strategically place the cotton on my face. The simplest lotion can do the magic of a rich serum if it's used in this way to make a lotion mask (see pp. 73–78). Likewise with facial scrub, which some people avoid because of its abrasiveness: the formula can be made milder and twice as effective by combining it with facial soap and warm water.

This is why I advise people to invest not money but care and attention in their skin.

I also encourage people to make the most of their palms and fingers. Warming a skincare product in your hands will help it to better penetrate the skin and double or even triple its effectiveness. By wrapping your hands around your face, the cosmetic and your own heat will act together like a steam iron, making your skin remarkably smooth. You can use your fingers to apply pressure, to push particles through pores to deliver them deep into your skin and improve circulation, or to massage your face and smooth out creases.

These are all inexpensive techniques that don't cost a single extra penny.

As sophisticated and quick-acting as today's beauty products may be, these virtues will go to waste if they're used in a slapdash way. So my advice to you is *Put your heart into every drop of the skincare products you choose.* Approaching your daily skincare routine with enthusiasm, urging your brown spots to disappear or your cheeks not to sag, will make a much greater difference than blindly spending a fortune on cosmetics.

Take in beauty with all your senses

My late husband used to tell me that I should expose myself to things of genuine quality. The two of us would often visit museums and view historic masterpieces, dine a couple times a month at fancy restaurants, or travel to foreign countries, where we'd be moved by sights of nature and streetscapes we had never seen before.

When you get out and about and experience new things, you're bound to feel as if the cells of your entire body are imbibing the essence of beauty, making you more beautiful. The face of someone who shuts herself up in a gloomy room all day is likely to be dull and impassive, while that of someone who goes outside and appreciates the beautiful things around her will naturally be expressive and content.

What is it that defines a woman's beauty? There are some who don't impress me with womanly charm in spite of their pretty faces, and others who somehow shine out in a crowd even though there's nothing particularly dazzling about them. I think of the actress Audrey Hepburn, whom I've always admired, as being one such woman with a special presence that transcended her natural beauty. She proved that even the wrinkles and sagging that come with age can be attractive just as they are, if they are part of the self-confidence and character of a woman who has lived life well. The wrinkles on such women appear not as signs of aging, but as marks of honor.

Don't fuss over every spot and line on your face. It isn't as if their presence diminishes your worth as a woman. Most brown spots and lines can be erased with patience, and, at any rate, the overall demeanor and luster of your face are far more important in determining the impression you give.

Of course, it's nice to have good skin—which is why I've carefully attended to my face through the years. But keep in mind that flawless skin isn't everything. Beauty isn't something to be plastered on from the outside; it's fake unless it also exudes from within.

I'm grateful to this day to my husband for having taught me to appreciate quality. Today, I take the time to surround my home with flowers, a love of mine. Sometimes I relax to the scent of incense or the sound of water, or enjoy my favorite music as it flows through the room. Then I feel my face soften, regardless of how tired I am, and I begin to feel beautiful.

So go out to a museum or park, or even just go window-shopping at a department store. No matter how busy you might be, and especially if you're working so hard you find yourself growing edgy, try to squeeze in some time for yourself—even if it's just one hour a month—to enjoy the beauty of life.

Make the mirror your ally

Every cosmetics counter and beauty salon has a mirror. Yet many women lack the courage to look their reflection in the face, perhaps because the presence of other people makes them self-conscious. And even when they do look at themselves, it's the flaws that seem to catch their eye: how wrinkled their faces are, how parched and flaky their skin is.

For such women, I offer this advice: *In the solitude of your own home, take a good, close look at your reflection every day.* In addition to choosing which cosmetics to use that day to improve your skin's condition, compliment yourself. For instance, if you gave yourself a face pack yesterday and your skin is in top shape, go ahead and marvel at it. Indulging in a bit of self-praise will do much good for your beauty. Again, don't be too opinionated about what's wrong with your face. As so often happens, the part of it that you like the least can be exactly what others find the most charming.

So, instead of hiding what you consider to be your flaw, try looking upon it as your unique feature and show it off. Imagine a plump woman who wears baggy clothing to cover up her curves: her efforts only call attention to her chubbiness. On the other hand, if the same woman wears form-fitting clothing instead, she'll enhance the attractiveness of her hips and breasts by putting their shapeliness into relief.

Many women make comments about how they'd love to have

a nose like this actress or how they wish they'd been born with big eyes like that celebrity. These are nothing but empty wishes. It's a wonderful thing to have a woman you look up to, but her way of life, her bearing, or her words and deeds are what make her so fascinating. Each face is different from the next, and it's a waste of time wanting to look like someone else.

In the final analysis, as I see it, a beautiful person is someone who knows herself inside and out and is comfortable being herself.

The mirror faithfully reflects your image, for good or for ill. Make an ally of it in your quest for self-refinement by keeping it with you at all times, viewing yourself objectively, just as you might check your reflection in a shop window.

Book time for yourself, not beauty salons

The other day someone asked me, "You treat your clients' skin every day at the salon as a skin beautician, but who looks after yours?"

The answer is, nobody.

I've never once been to a beauty salon in private, the reason being that I can take care of my own skin. Now, you may think I'm special. After all, I used to work as the manager of the Christian Dior salon in Tokyo, and I still treat clients at my own salon on a daily basis. The fact is, though, you can perform self-treatments exactly as I do if you just get the hang of it. Anyone can

Women often blame their unkempt skin on lack of money and time. They have all kinds of excuses.

"I'm so busy looking after the kids, I don't have any time."

"I don't have the money to go to a salon."

Truth be told, once you read my book, you'll realize you can achieve beauty without spending much time or money, and you needn't rely on a salon to do it.

In this book, I'll share with you self-care techniques you can use to perfect your skin with your own hands—tricks that involve no special equipment, can be done easily in the bath or living room, and are just as effective as the treatments given at a salon. The only items you need are cotton, plastic wrap, ice, and a few basic cosmetics (see Getting Started, pp. 23–29). And the best implements of all, of course, are your own palms and fingers.

Start out by finding just five minutes of time for yourself each day to free your senses and care for your skin. You'll feel your mind and body being soothed much more deeply than you would at an expensive salon.

Gear down in times of trouble

Here's something I've repeated over and over to cosmetics addicts: *If you want good skin, have the courage to cut back on cosmetics.*

My first book, *Saeki Chizu no tayoruna keshohin!* (Chizu Saeki's "Don't Rely on Cosmetics!") was subtitled *Kao o arau no o oyame nasai!* (Stop Washing Your Face!). Upon first glance at that subtitle, a lot of people might question my sanity, particularly in Japan where it's considered common sense to wash the face twice, first with cleanser, then with facial soap. So what on earth was I saying?

My motto is that excessive care damages the skin. Being alive, skin is equipped with a self-cleansing mechanism, and pampering it too much only weakens that ability. Basic care is of course essential—things like guarding against UV rays before going outside and cooling down your skin with lotion after a day of sports and sweat. But washing your face several times over because you have oily skin, or daubing your face with pricey cream because your skin is dry, is just bad for your skin.

If your skin is crying out for help, now is the time to sit down and take a no-nonsense look at it—like a doctor interviewing a patient—to discern what it really needs and what it doesn't. Although people with problem skin are tempted to try all sorts of remedies, taking a break is what they should be doing. Sometimes less is more.

The ultimate skincare I recommend is what I call "skin fasting." The essence of the routine is simple: don't do anything. I don't mean that you should allow your skin to fall into a constant state of neglect. Rather, decide on one day a week to do nothing more than rinse your face. This will reawaken your skin's innate strength and bring it back to health.

I suggest skin fasting because, having seen the skin of many women, I've learned that the skin condition of those who use too many products is far worse than that of those who use nothing at all. In short, this is the perfect way to break away from the addiction to cosmetics that so many women today fall victim to.

As you will have realized by now, the fundamentals of skincare are surprisingly simple. There's no need to go through an entire regimen that's longer than you can remember.

In addition to treatment, I also provide counseling to my salon clients. I occasionally ask clients to bring in all of the cosmetic products they currently use so I can take a look at them. Most people have a heap of products they don't need, and essentials only amount to half of what they own.

Try reviewing the contents of your cosmetic bag and reorganizing your inventory. You'll realize that your money will be better spent investing in what you really need than in buying a hodgepodge of products.

Learn from a linen handkerchief

There's a shop called Oshiro Lace in the Shimbashi district of Tokyo. I've always been fond of the shop's handkerchiefs, and I often give them to people as a token of thanks. The pure white linen handkerchiefs with embroidered initials—also in white— are lovely, and everyone is delighted with the gift.

By the way, have you ever wondered why babies have such smooth skin? It's because their skin hasn't been exposed to UV rays or dryness—much like the condition of a brand-new white handkerchief. Unused white handkerchiefs are crisply starched and spotless, without a single thread out of place. This is like the perfection of fresh, resilient baby skin.

After being repeatedly washed and dried, though, the once-white handkerchief will grow faded and worn. It will also become spotted and wrinkly with use.

How the handkerchief will fare is really up to its owner. An owner determined to make it last will gently hand-wash it when it's dirty, bleach it when yellowed, and iron it out when it gets wrinkled. A linen handkerchief can remain clean and usable for a long time if you take good care of it. On the other hand, if you give up on it and let it sit for a long time all crumpled because it's stained anyway, the handkerchief will never regain its former beauty.

Skincare is similar in many ways because human skin is, after all, a fabric of sorts. You can erase brown spots by applying vitamin C serum, smooth out lines by hydrating and stretching them, and brighten your skin when it's dull by washing it with scrub. By steadfastly looking after your skin in this way, you'll be able to keep it looking fresh as a brand-new linen handkerchief for decades. To further the analogy, going to a beauty salon or investing in intensive treatment is like taking your handkerchief to a costly dry cleaner's.

My advice: *If you want your skin to stay beautiful forever, care for it just as you would your cherished possessions*.

Don't overfeed your skin

With the Westernization of the Japanese diet, obesity is on the rise in Japan. Consequently, even young people nowadays are suffering from what were once known as adult afflictions—now called lifestyle diseases—such as high blood pressure and arteriosclerosis.

I love good food, and ordering various foods from across Japan has become one of my favorite diversions. But I never eat in large quantities; I just enjoy small amounts of truly delicious food. Thanks to this habit, I've never grown obese, and I enjoy perfectly good health.

A lot of people don't know that you can also overfeed your skin. Looking back on the women I've met up to now, those with skin problems generally do just that: overfeed their skin. Their skin is in a state of skin obesity, as it were. Bombarded with so many different products, a person's skin often launches an ugly protest. Noting this, the person thinks something must be done, and applies rich creams, further impairing the skin's natural ability to clean itself.

To avoid this vicious cycle, I make a point of telling people to look at their skin and touch it before putting anything on it. Take a good look at your skin in the mirror, and carefully pick out and use only the products you really need. By doing so, you'll keep from acquiring lifestyle diseases of the skin.

If your skin is dry, for instance, you may be apt to spread cream on your face. But upon closer observation, you'll notice that what the skin is craving above all is moisture. You should first amply hydrate it with lotion and serum, and only then seal it with cream.

Think of it this way: you wouldn't take a withering potted tree and dump concentrated fertilizer on it. The first thing you'd do, rather, is give it plenty of water and make way for the nutrients to seep into the soil. The skin is no different.

Skincare products are food for the skin, so I advise you to avoid overfeeding it. Just as a once-obese person who has shaken off extra weight may discover renewed confidence and freedom of movement, skin will also start to feel better, and look better, once it's no longer buried in cosmetics.

Food and water will transform the skin in three months

Dieting is very popular these days, but my belief is that you should eat if you want to be beautiful. After all, the human body is made up of the food and drink we take in orally. You can't hope for skin beauty if you use luxurious cosmetics but eat junk food all the time. According to nutritional science, the cells of the body are renewed roughly every three months; in effect, it is your daily meals that create your future body.

Every day, I make a point of consuming vitamin- and mineral-rich vegetables and fruits, as well as beans and dairy products with their proteins and dietary fibers. I also drink a good 1.5 liters of water daily. The key is to eat in a balanced manner, rather than just one food at a time, such as just bread or just meat. Nutritional balance is also important for efficiently burning off the calories you've taken in with the bread or meat.

In Japan, we have a custom of saying "Itadakimasu," roughly meaning "I gratefully receive this," while putting our palms together in a position of prayer before beginning a meal. We do this to humbly thank the organisms of the plant and animal kingdoms that we are about to consume for the sake of our physical well-being. Gratitude is very important for achieving beauty. In the same way, I thank my skin every day during my skincare routine. In response, the skin will be gratified and increase its beauty.

CHAPTER 1

Getting Started

A short list of essential tools
and cosmetics.

Tools

Saeki-style skincare requires no exclusive products. In my experience, it's hard to continuously use expensive products or ones that you can only buy at select stores. Inexpensive products, on the other hand—and ones that are readily available—can be used every day without much deliberation, and are therefore good for your mental as well as your physical hygiene.

What you need to have on hand are everyday household products—cotton swabs, plastic wrap, shower caps, and so on. The only exception is cotton squares. While cotton is widely available in most drugstores, only 100% natural, absorbent cotton will work with my lotion-mask technique. And ideally, I recommend thick cotton that you can pull apart into layers.

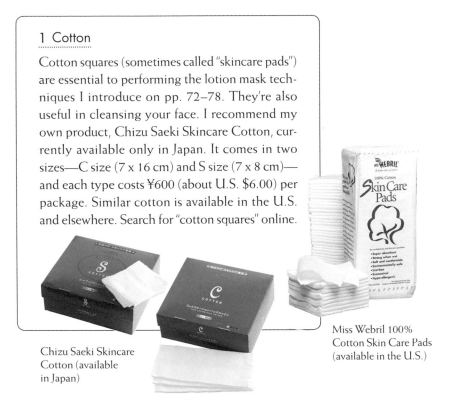

1 Cotton

Cotton squares (sometimes called "skincare pads") are essential to performing the lotion mask techniques I introduce on pp. 72–78. They're also useful in cleansing your face. I recommend my own product, Chizu Saeki Skincare Cotton, currently available only in Japan. It comes in two sizes—C size (7 x 16 cm) and S size (7 x 8 cm)—and each type costs ¥600 (about U.S. $6.00) per package. Similar cotton is available in the U.S. and elsewhere. Search for "cotton squares" online.

Miss Webril 100% Cotton Skin Care Pads (available in the U.S.)

Chizu Saeki Skincare Cotton (available in Japan)

2 Towels

No skincare regimen is complete without towels and washcloths. Make sure the ones you use are 100% cotton. See pp. 106–11 for the use of towels in hot and cool treatments.

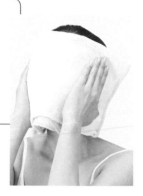

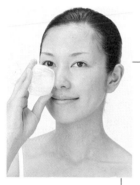

3 Ice or cool packs

Ice is an essential ingredient of the cool treatment I outline on pp. 109–11. I recommend large ice cubes. Making them is easy: simply freeze water in empty yogurt containers or plastic cups. Cool packs may also be used.

4 Plastic wrap

You can wrap plastic wrap around your face and arms to create a sauna-like environment that will improve your skin's health and shine. Be sure to use strong wrap that sticks well, rather than the flimsier kind.

5 Shower caps

A shower cap over your face, with breathing holes cut out, can achieve the same sauna-effect as plastic wrap. But who wants to take a big roll of plastic wrap on vacation or a business trip? See pp. 104–05 for the Instant Steam Pack technique.

6 Swan-neck squeeze bottle

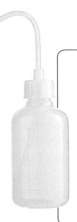

Squeeze bottles of this sort can generally be found in art or tattoo supply stores, or online (search for "Nalgene wash bottles" or "germicidal squeeze bottles"). I use them for water massages (pp. 112–13). The exact shape of the dispenser isn't that important, as long as it can be used to squirt a steady stream of water.

7 Your own hands and fingers

Your hands and fingers are the ultimate tools. You can use them to wash and massage your face, as well as examine it to understand your skin's needs. You can also use them to warm up cosmetics and to apply creams, serums, and liquid foundation. As you'll see, your hands have the power to heal weak or damaged skin, and you should use that power to its fullest.

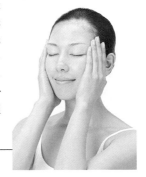

Saeki-style skincare essentials ❷

Cosmetics

It's not much use having a jumble of expensive cosmetics without knowledge of what each one does or how it should be applied. Be sure to understand the purpose of each product you buy, and use it correctly, putting your full heart into each step. Remember to warm the product in your hands before applying it—doing so will greatly enhance its effectiveness.

Here are some of the basic skincare products I use. Note that these are only examples; choose what suits you best after trying out various products on your own skin.

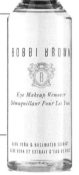

1 Makeup remover

Take special care to completely remove the makeup around your eyes. Residual eye shadow or mascara pigments can lead to dullness and wrinkles.

Bobbi Brown Eye Makeup Remover

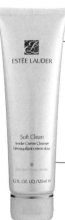

2 Cleanser

My skincare policy focuses more on the removal of makeup than on its application, so be choosy with cleanser. A cream-type cleanser is best for those over 30.

Estée Lauder Soft Clean
Tender Crème Cleanser

3 Facial scrub

The skin has a shedding cycle of 28 days, but the dead cells can remain there longer if metabolism is slow. Help your skin exfoliate by washing with scrub once or twice a week.

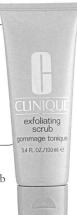

Clinique Exfoliating Scrub

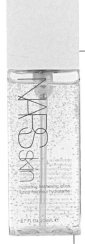

NARSskin Hydrating Freshening Lotion

4 Lotion

A key part of my skincare program is the lotion mask (pp. 73–78). Though involving only lotion, water, and cotton, it works miracles. Lotions—not to be confused with toners or astringents—condition your skin surface. There are basically two types: hydrating lotions and brightening lotions. The ingredients are typically 80% water and 10% alcohol, along with an assortment of moisturizing agents and therapeutic ingredients. I strongly recommend only those lotions that contain little or no alcohol.

5 Serum

Serum is like a nutritional supplement, penetrating deep into your skin and energizing it from within. There are all kinds of serums available—brightening serums, hydrating serums, vitamin C serums, and so on—so choose one that best suits your skin's needs.

Estée Lauder Advanced Night Repair Protective Recovery Complex

6 Eye cream

The area around the eyes is prone to dryness, and the muscles there get worn down on a daily basis. Use eye cream to revitalize the skin in this area.

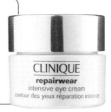

Clinique Repairwear
Intensive Eye Cream

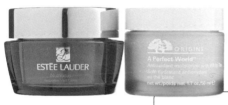

Origins A Perfect World™
Antioxidant Moisturizer

Estée Lauder Nutritious
Restorative Night Cream

7 Emulsion or cream

These products serve as "lids" to seal in the serum's nutrients. If cream is the lid of a pressure cooker, then emulsion is a lighter glass lid. Cream rather than emulsion is advisable for those over 30 because it's stronger and better at keeping in moisture, which we tend to lose with age.

8 Sunscreen

There are two types of sunscreen: gentler types that reflect UV rays with scattering agents, and those containing absorbing agents to keep the rays from getting past the surface. I recommend using sunscreen in your daily skincare routine all year round.

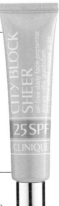

Clinique City Block
Sheer Oil-free Daily Face
Protector SPF 25

CHAPTER 2

Skincare Basics & Massage Techniques

Simply touching or pressing
your face with your fingers and palms,
or wrapping your hands around it,
will do wonders for your skin.

Polish your skin inside and out

The most magnificent flower exposes only a small portion of its existence to view. It can blossom beautifully because its roots spread underground, pumping up water and nutrients with all their might.

Our skin, too, is only partially visible, and what happens on the inside is just as vital as what we can see on the outside.

Loosely speaking, human skin is made up of the epidermis and dermis. What we normally call "skin" is the epidermis, or surface skin—the layer that we can see. The dermis, or true skin, is the layer that supports the epidermis; this is what corresponds to a flower's roots. Crisscrossing fibers in the dermis lift up the epidermis above by retaining moisture and nutrients, giving skin its healthy resilience.

When we're young, the healthy fibers of our skin hold plenty of moisture and nutrients. But with age, the fibrous structures shrivel. Our skin then becomes prone to dryness and malnutrition and, having lost its elasticity, grows paper-thin. This is what results in wrinkles and age spots.

Serums rescue your skin from this predicament; they reach into the depths of the skin to nourish and invigorate it. So if you're past the age of 30, I strongly recommend that you use serum regularly. Looking after your surface skin won't be enough, especially once you begin noticing sagging or lines on your face. Let's examine the skin from the outside in.

Epidermal care

The epidermis is the surface part of the skin. Smoothness and firmness, qualities that define the texture of your skin, will be lost if you don't give this layer due attention. Take good care of your epidermis by regularly applying lotion masks (pp. 73–78), exfoliating dead surface cells, protecting it from UV rays, and cleansing it properly.

Dermal care

Between the epidermis and the dermis is the dermal-epidermal junction, and below this is the dermis. The dermis determines the youthfulness of your skin—its moisture and resilience. Serums are what pump energy into the aging dermis. They pass through the epidermis into the dermal layer, plumping out the fibrous structures made of substances such as collagen and elastin.

Structure of the skin

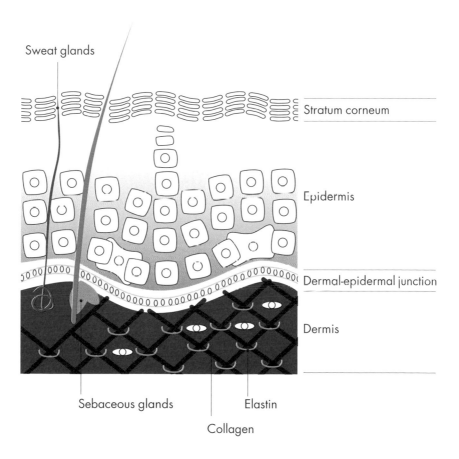

Our skin basically consists of the epidermis and dermis, and the dermal-epidermal junction connects the two. Old epidermal cells rise to the surface to form the stratum corneum, or horny layer. This outer layer should be shed once a week using facial scrub.

Look, touch, ask

The first step to achieving beautiful skin is getting to know your face. As immaculate as your skin may be, your face is bound to give others the sense that something is not quite right if it is distorted or sagging. There are three basic ways to self-check your face: look, touch, and ask. Make this a daily habit.

First, scan your face in the mirror for sagging and distortion. If you notice that the corner of your right eye is lower than that of your left, the right side of your face is sagging. Tone the muscles on the right by making a conscious effort to chew on that side. By "correcting" imperfections in your face, you can bring it closer to symmetry, one of the basic requisites for beauty.

The three "corners" of the face

Look at your face head-on and check for any drooping in the three corners of your face—the corners of the eyebrows, eyes, and mouth. The side with more drooping will begin sagging first.

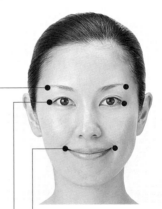

Corners of the eyebrows

Corners of the eyes   Corners of the mouth

The clown smile

Smile at the mirror like a clown, with lips closed and corners lifted. If one side of your face gets furrowed more deeply than the other, that side is slacker. Fix it by consciously adjusting your chewing habits and sleeping position: chew on that side of your mouth, and sleep on that side of your face. With little efforts like these, you can make your face more symmetrical.

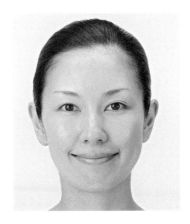

Your present, past, and future faces

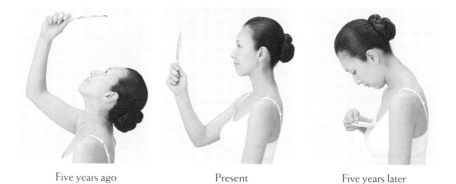

Five years ago   Present   Five years later

See how your face changes when you look at it in a hand mirror held directly above, in front of, and below your face. You need to take good care of your skin to turn back the clock five years.

The five goals of skin beauty

Every morning, as soon as I get up, I look in the mirror to inspect my face: Are my cheeks dry? Is my skin looking dull? Are there circles under my eyes? At the same time, I also assess how I can make myself look better.

It helps to have a clear idea of what sort of skin you want to have rather than haphazardly going about your skincare. Oddly enough, many people are not certain just what healthy, beautiful skin is. In answer to this problem, I created important criteria for defining beautiful skin, based on the experience I gained back in my days working in the cosmetics industry. I call these the five goals of skin beauty: moisture, smoothness, firmness, elasticity, and clear complexion. The ideal skin is one that possesses all of these qualities.

With this five-point evaluation system, all you have to do is identify the areas where your skin needs work, and move toward balancing out the five qualities. This is where caring for both your epidermis and dermis comes into play. Smoothness and firmness are primarily achieved through epidermal care, while dermal care is the key to moisture, elasticity, and complexion.

Moisture

Skin that meets this goal . . .

1 Has a balanced oil and moisture content

2 Allows smooth application of makeup

3 Has a moist and velvety texture

4 Is springy to the touch

5 Has clarity

In drought circumstances, the ground can become so dry that water runs off its surface. However, once tilled and hydrated, earth becomes rich, soft, and able to absorb moisture. In much the same way, human skin softens up and plumps out when it's richly hydrated, and becomes more receptive to skincare products.

Your skin craves moisture if your face is greasy and yet peeling around the eyes and mouth, if your complexion isn't clear, or if your makeup won't stay on. If you notice any of these, you should focus on hydrating your skin, not on removing oil. Lotion masks (pp. 73–78), water massages (pp. 112–13), moisturizing serums, and full-bodied creams will help.

In addition, dryness can cause lines and wrinkles. Guard against dehydration by frequently dabbing eye cream around your eyes, an area that's particularly susceptible to drying.

Moisture check

Do the palms of your hands stick to your cheeks?

Firmly press your hands to your cheeks, with thumbs against the hollows behind your earlobes. Slowly let go. If you feel the cheek skin sticking to the palms of your hands, it's a sign that your skin is moist. Those with insufficient moisture most likely have thin, dryness-prone skin, and the skin around the mouth and eyes may be powdery or peeling.

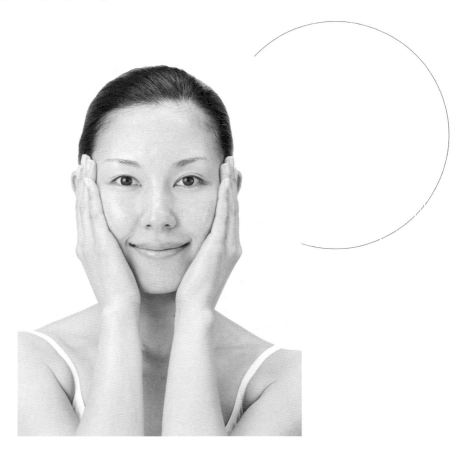

Smoothness

Skin that meets this goal . . .

1 Is soft

2 Has an even texture

3 Retains makeup well

4 Produces relatively little oil

5 Has an active metabolism

Fine-textured, smooth skin is born through a healthy metabolism and regular replacement of skin cells. If your skin is perpetually thickened with unshed dead cells, or if oil production is excessive, there's little hope for fine skin.

The top priority for smooth skin is to make sure dirt doesn't linger in your pores. Clean your face especially carefully in those areas where dirt and oil tend to clog the pores—the forehead, the chin, and the wings of the nose.

Replenishing moisture is key to regulating oil production. Some good ways of doing this are treating your face with a lotion mask (pp. 73–78) and applying moisturizing serum to the areas where the pores clog easily. Also, you can help speed up your skin's shedding cycle by using scrub or face packs two or three times a week.

Lack of sleep, psychological stress, and an unbalanced diet are all factors that can contribute to excessive oil. Try to stay relaxed in mind and body and maintain a balanced diet for your skin and well-being.

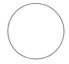

Smoothness check

Do your forehead and nose have a modest amount of oil?

You have smooth skin if there's a modest amount of oil on your fingertips after touching your nose and forehead. If your fingertips get greasy, your skin is probably hardened and has a rough texture. The cause is excessive oil production. Exfoliate the T-zone once or twice a week using scrub. People with oily skin tend to wash their faces too hard, but overwashing only leads to more oil. Try to balance the moisture and oil content of your skin by giving it lotion masks and water massages.

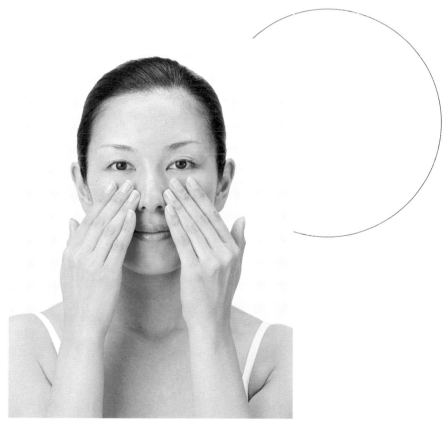

Firmness

Skin that meets this goal . . .

1 Springs back when pressed with the fingers

2 Is fresh and glowing

3 Has an excellent balance of oil and moisture

4 Feels moist

5 Has few lines and wrinkles

Firm skin can also be described as skin with luster. I think of the word "lustrous" as being the ultimate compliment for a woman's skin.

Firmness is lost when the skin falls short on all three counts of moisture, oil, and nutrients, or when its metabolism is sluggish. To improve firmness, make a habit of applying treatment creams and face packs that will help provide these needed components. Also, actively use serums to plump out your skin from deep down in the dermal fibers.

Dust, air conditioning, and UV rays are all archenemies of your skin. Before going out, be sure to put on day cream to protect your skin from these perils, as they can result in dry or tired skin that lacks firmness and luster.

Foods that can improve firmness include meat, fish, and dairy products, as they include proteins to boost cellular activity within the skin. Foods rich in vitamin C can also help.

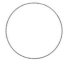

Firmness check

Do fine lines stand out when you lightly pull your skin outward?

With thumbs behind the earlobes and the other fingers over the temples, gently pull your facial skin outward. If vertical lines form around the eyes, or if you have deep wrinkles, it's proof that your skin is giving out in the deep dermal layer and losing firmness. Make sure to use serum and cream, which will provide your skin with moisture, oil, and nutrients, in your morning and evening care. It's also a good idea to incorporate epidermal care, such as face packs and scrubs. Beware of too much washing.

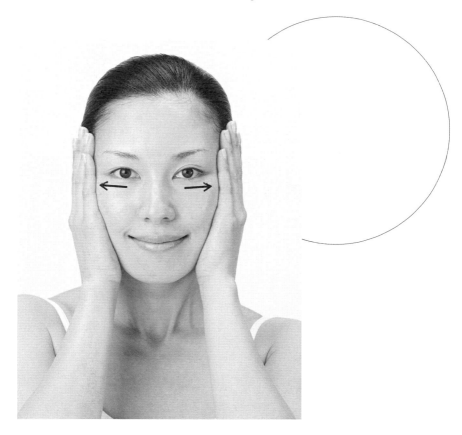

Elasticity

Skin that meets this goal . . .

1 Is springy when pressed with the fingers

2 Has radiance and glow

3 Has a fine and plump texture

4 Shows minimal sagging around the corners of the eyes and mouth

5 Is moist overall

The skin we all have as babies, soft yet resilient as a rubber ball, gradually diminishes in elasticity with age for a number of reasons. The cells of the epidermis grow lean and flat, the fibers of the dermis turn hard and brittle and lose their ability to regenerate, and skin metabolism slows down.

Reduced elasticity, in turn, will bring on a variety of changes, such as less definition of the facial contour, loose skin around the eyes and mouth, and fine wrinkles.

What's key to keeping these symptoms at bay is dermal care; you can't get rid of the sag without mending the substructure that supports the epidermis. Use serum day and night to strengthen the skin's fibers. After refining its texture with a lotion mask (pp. 73–78), further feed it with moisture and oil by applying serum (pp. 79–81). And remember to exfoliate your skin once a week.

Skin that has lost its elasticity produces a tired impression and can make you look older. Restore your skin's vigor by generously fortifying both the epidermal and dermal layers.

Elasticity check

Can you pinch plenty of cheek flesh?
Does the pinching hurt?

When you pinch your cheeks with the thumb and forefinger of each hand, is the flesh between the fingers thicker on one side? Does the pinching hurt? You will not be able to pinch a thick bit of flesh, nor will the pinching hurt, if the skin has a worn-out dermis and low elasticity. This skin type is thin, with visible veins, and will not bounce back when pressed with the fingers. Fortify the dermal fibers by using serums enriched with collagen and elastin. Before going to bed, supply the needed oil with a moist cream. Also, try to chew equally on both sides, since chewing habits can affect skin elasticity.

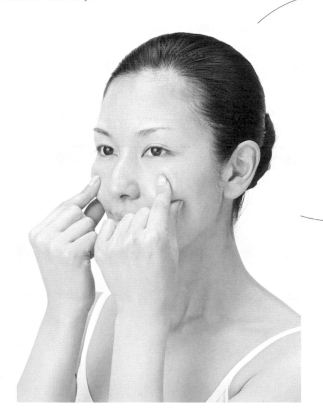

Clear complexion

Skin that meets this goal . . .

1 Is soft and firm

2 Is moist overall

3 Has clarity

4 Has an active metabolism

5 Gives the impression of vitality

Skin with a good complexion makes a woman look healthy and young, as well as enhancing the effect of makeup. While physical wellness is of course one factor affecting the condition of your skin, many other hazards can ruin its clarity and complexion, such as dead cells clinging to the surface and thickening the skin, darkening and dryness caused by UV rays, mental stress, lack of sleep, and an unbalanced diet.

Things to work toward in your lifestyle should include avoiding stress and consciously consuming vitamin C in your diet. In terms of skincare, it's crucial to protect your skin from UV rays and air conditioning by wearing day cream, to exfoliate once or twice weekly, and to invigorate your dermis with serum.

Nowadays you can also find skincare products with aromatherapeutic effects. Incorporating products with relaxing aromas in your evening skincare regimen may be a good idea, too.

Smoking and excessive drinking can result in a sallow complexion, so try to remember that moderation, at least, is vital for your beauty and health.

Complexion check

Do you feel warmth when you place your fingers beneath your eyes?

Place your fingers beneath the eyes and slide them back and forth twice between the nose and temples. You have a healthy complexion if your skin feels warm after doing this. If not, your skin most likely has a thick layer of dead cells, looks dull, and is prone to problems. The primary causes are a dehydrated epidermis and a slow metabolism, which keeps your skin from shedding old cells. Effective remedies include exfoliating once or twice a week with facial scrub and applying serum that clarifies your skin. In addition, give yourself lymph massages (pp. 53–59) to drain out waste matter, and drink plenty of water to improve blood flow.

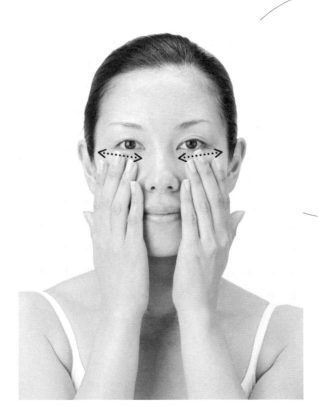

Six Saeki-style massage techniques

I'm now going to share with you six kinds of massages practiced by professionals. These are massages I've used for many years. Each movement has meaning, so I advise you to try these out with a proper understanding of their purpose, rather than mindlessly following the directions.

Though many people may picture circling hand movements and other complex motions when they think of massages, the techniques illustrated here are all very simple—things like pressing your hands against your cheeks or wrapping your face with your hands to warm it up. But keep in mind that these massages won't be half as effective if you focus on just the surface skin.

Once again, it's helpful to remember that the epidermis is only the outermost layer of your skin, and there's no use caring for your epidermis unless you take care of what's underneath it at the same time. It's the same with clothing: when your muscles are in shape, anything you wear looks better.

If you take a sip of water, it will simply stay in your mouth. It won't go in any further and be useful to you unless you have the strength to swallow—unless you use your muscles to do so. By the same token, your skin won't take in nutrients if the dermal layer isn't in good shape. That's why my skincare approach consists of double care—polishing the epidermis on the one hand and toning the dermis and muscles underneath on the other. Massages are what tone the dermis and muscles. Think of these routines as improving your skin's basic fitness.

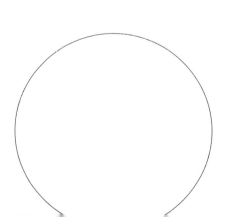

1 Stretching techniques

These are basic, caressing massages that can be performed at various points in a skincare routine.

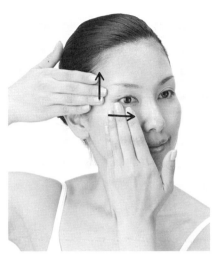

With the fingertips, stretch the skin under your eye inward while lifting the temple skin with your other hand.

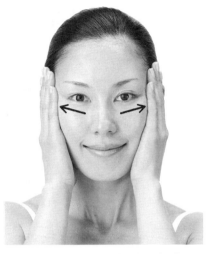

Hold your cheeks in your hands and pull your whole face outward with some pressure.

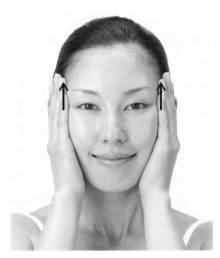

Lift the facial skin upward with your fingers or hands.

2 Pushing & pulling techniques

These are somewhat stronger than the stretches introduced above. They'll help cosmetics sink in better and improve lymph flow (see p. 54).

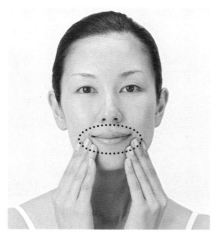

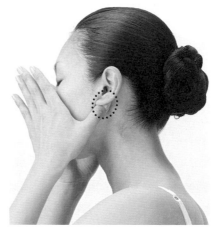

Gently press the skin around the lips and the corners of your mouth, where lymph nodes are concentrated.

Waste tends to accumulate in the lymph nodes behind the ears. Press that area with the balls of your thumbs to help the waste flow downward.

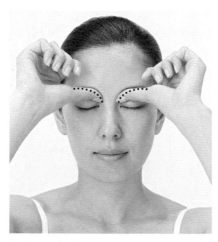

Push into the hollows beneath the eyebrows, another area with many lymph nodes, using the balls of your thumbs.

3 Pinching & lifting techniques

These are instrumental in remedying lines and sagging. They can also help correct muscular habits.

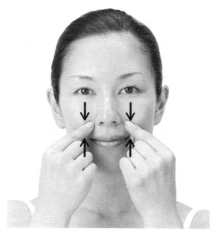

Pinch the laugh lines vertically and press outward with the balls of your fingers.

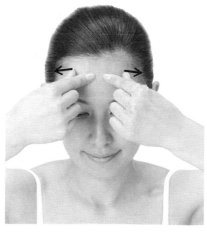

For forehead wrinkles, pinch the skin with your fingertips and ease the muscles from the center toward your temples.

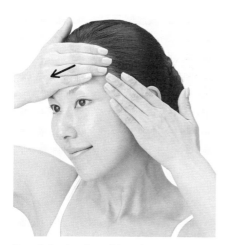

Stretch forehead wrinkles sideways with one hand while holding your temple in place with the other.

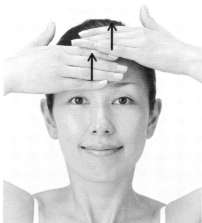

The muscles of your forehead will sag just as its skin will. Pull the muscles upward with alternating hands.

4 The piano touch

This massage is for areas around the eyes and mouth with thin, delicate skin. The idea is to massage your skin as if playing the piano.

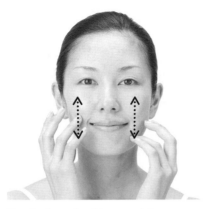

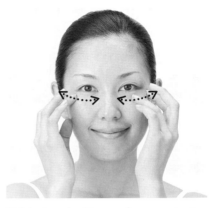

Gently drum the skin around the corners of your mouth and cheeks to lift the muscles, firming your face.

Lightly drum the skin around your eyes to stimulate circulation and attenuate fine wrinkles.

5 Jiggling techniques

These are highly relaxing. The idea is to jiggle your scalp and facial skin with both hands.

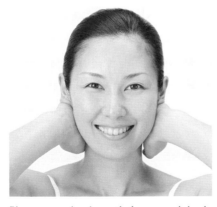

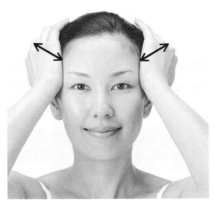

Place your palms beneath the ears and slowly move them back and forth to improve lymph flow.

Press your palms against the temples and gently jiggle the skin under your hands for a relaxing effect.

6 Pressing techniques

These are massages that act on the dermis. They will deliver warmth to it, thereby improving circulation and giving your face a healthy color.

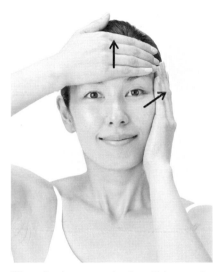 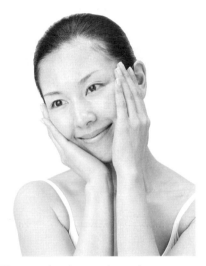

Warm the skin as you slowly pull the muscles in different directions, outward and upward.

Wrap your hands around your face to warm the skin.

BEAUTY COLUMN

Skin fasting—the ultimate care

I once had the experience of fasting at a health institute. I began feeling queasy about two days into the fast, the culprit apparently being the food additives I'd been consuming every day. After my digestive system had been purged, though, I felt cleansed in both mind and body—literally detoxified.

The skin gets worn out by a daily diet of cosmetics, too. So I advise people to give their skin a day of rest once a week. I call it skin fasting, the idea being to let your skin spend a whole day free of makeup and skincare products to heighten its natural healing power. It's the ultimate care, a kind of R&R for your skin.

Doing a water massage (pp. 112–13) beforehand will enhance the effect of the fast. Loosen the underlying muscles with the natural force of water and awaken your skin's innate strength, then go to bed without applying anything on your face. You'll get more out of your beauty sleep this way, jump-starting the process of regeneration. The skin, after all, has the ability to cleanse itself without loads of pampering, so every once in a while, help your skin recuperate by just letting it be.

CHAPTER 3

Lymph
Massages

Doing these massages daily while
sitting in the bath, watching TV,
or just before applying makeup
will make your skin grow lustrous.

Refreshen your complexion with lymph massages

Our bodies have a network of lymph vessels, much like the blood vessels of the circulatory system. What flows through this network, carrying away pathogens, microscopic foreign particles, and the waste of dead cells, is lymph fluid. Foreign bodies, toxins, and other waste products are filtered out from the fluid at lymph nodes distributed throughout the network.

Lymph massages are a great way to enhance the workings of this lymphatic system. Sluggish lymph flow will cause toxins to build up and make your face look puffy. To reverse this, you need to detoxify your system by draining the toxins into the nodes. If cleansing your face is the first step in surface care, the first in subsurface care—basic to achieving healthy skin—is cleansing your body from under the skin by flushing out the waste in your lymph vessels.

Accordingly, when I begin a facial treatment, I don't even think about the surface skin; lymph massages come first. I facilitate the draining of waste matter by carefully massaging the collarbones and neck and then pressing the lymph nodes in the armpits. This bit of extra effort, which you can perform for yourself, will tighten your face and miraculously improve the luster of your skin.

I encourage you to get into the habit of doing lymph massages before starting any other element of your skincare routine.

Lymph node pressure points for fresh skin

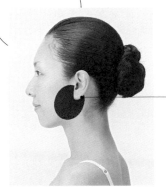

Behind the ears (parotid lymph nodes)

The parotid glands, where the parotid lymph nodes are located, are actually in front of the ears, but part of them also lies behind them. The lymph nodes in the small hollows behind the ears affect facial swelling and firmness.

The sides of the neck (cervical lymph nodes)

These lymph nodes extend downward from under the ears.

Above the collarbones (supraclavicular lymph nodes)

These are located in the hollows above the collarbones.

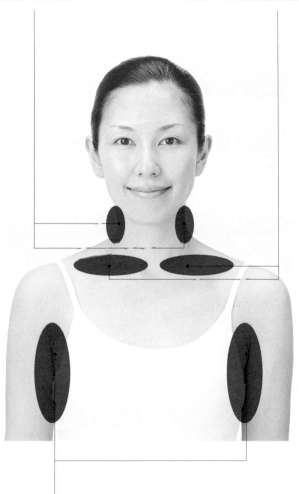

Armpits (axillary lymph nodes)

Lymph nodes in the armpits. This is where you'll drain the waste you've gathered from the face, neck, and collarbones.

Fight the double chin

Your facial contour will lose its definition when lymph flow is lazy around your ears and neck. To keep my face line from going soft and to prevent a double chin, I do this massage whenever I find the time.

Push the lymph fluids from the underside of your chin toward the ears by sliding your thumbs along your jaw. Firmly press the lymph nodes in the hollows behind your ears, then massage down the neck so as to drain the lymphatic waste toward the collar-bones.

By continuing this technique, you will find that sagging de-creases, and your face line will sharpen up in a few months.

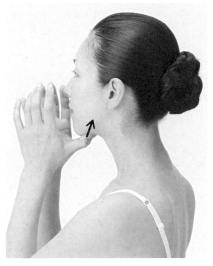

1 With both thumbs, massage the underside of your jaw from the point of your chin to-ward the ears.

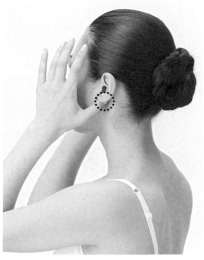

2 When you reach the ears, press the lymph nodes in the hollows behind them and push out the waste.

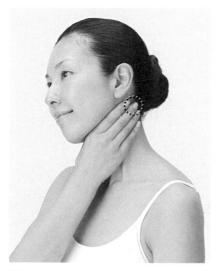

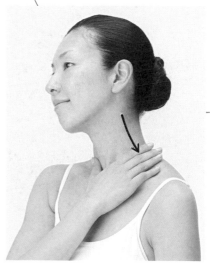

3 Press the lymph nodes under one ear with the fingers of your other hand while keeping your palm flush againt your neck.

4 Slide your hand downward so as to drain the waste to the collarbones. Repeat steps 3 and 4 for the other side of your neck.

Care for your neck

The neck is one part of your body that moves around more than you'd imagine—to and fro, up and down, twisting this way and that. For such an active area, though, its skin is surprisingly delicate and easily wrinkled. So after I take a bath, I make a point of caring for my neck before moving on to my face. A flabby neck also makes your face look big.

People often ask me if it's okay to use hand cream for the neck. My answer is no. Most neck creams are made to effectively firm your neck skin and increase its elasticity with vital collagen and elastin. They're a highly recommended addition to your dressing table, especially for those who are 30 years old or older.

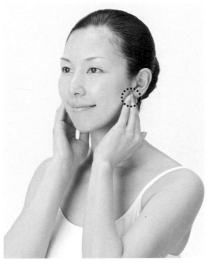 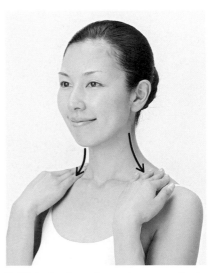

1 Take a generous amount of neck cream in your hands and press the lymph nodes under the ears with your middle fingers.

2 With the flats of your fingers, push the trapped waste down along the sides of your neck toward the collarbones.

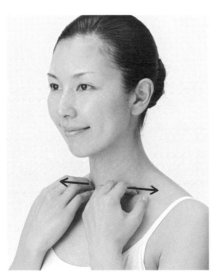

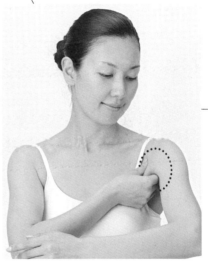

3 Insert your four fingers into the hollows above the collarbones and send the waste out toward your shoulders.

4 Drain the waste from the collarbones into the axillary lymph nodes under your arms, and finish off by pressing the armpits.

The elixir of imagination

When people ask me whether I'm lonely without my husband or whether I hope to find a new partner, I'm not exactly sure how to answer them. Why? Because I'm always falling in love. With men on screen, that is. I delight in these momentary movie star crushes, the best part of which is that I find myself in love with a different man every day.

It's often said that women are the most beautiful when they're in love. But you don't always bump into the right man at the right time, do you? Luckily for women, though, I've heard that even make-believe romances like mine are powerful enough to excite the secretion of female hormones.

I'm a master at fantasizing. When I cook, for example, I imagine who I'm having over for dinner and set the table for two even if I'm actually eating alone. Imagination is a valuable resource in many settings, especially when it gets your adrenaline pumping.

Imagination is also important when making up your face. Your application will come out a lot more nicely if you do it thinking about who you're going to see that day and how you'd like to look.

I like to capitalize on everything our bodies have to offer, from our hands and fingers to the warmth of touch. The hormones we produce are no exception. Adrenaline is, in a manner of speaking, our internal beauty serum. A bit of heart-throbbing excitement makes a great supplement for healthy skin.

CHAPTER 4

Everyday Skincare

Many women spend a fortune on beauty salons—but you can get similar results at home for a fraction of the cost.

Protection in the morning

In the morning, your main objective should be to protect your skin from the many perils awaiting it in the day ahead: UV rays, air conditioning, cigarette smoke, exhaust gases, and more.

Start out by checking your face in the mirror and deciding what it needs right now. Next, consider your schedule. Will you be outdoors? Or sitting for a long stretch in an air-conditioned room? Choose cosmetics to safeguard your skin according to what you'll be doing or where you'll be during the day.

Next, I advise you to warm the cosmetics in your hands before delivering them into your pores with your fingers. Your skin will absorb warmed products more readily, helping your makeup last longer.

Morning care

1 Washing
My method is to just rinse the face with lukewarm water in the morning. If you wish to use facial soap, lather it well, wrap your face in the foam, then rinse thoroughly.

2 Lotion
Applying lotion with your hands is fine, but a lotion mask (pp. 73–78) will refresh your skin even better, in just three minutes.

3 Serum
Feel free to choose different serums according to your skin's condition. I use deep-penetrating serums to nourish the dermis.

4 Emulsion/ cream
Emulsions and creams seal in the nutrients you've just given your skin. Be sure to warm them in your hands first.

5 Primer
Choose the right primer for your day's plans, such as one with sun protection or skin-brightening features. It can be either a thick cream or a lighter emulsion.

6 Foundation
I recommend liquid foundation for those over 30. By carefully working the foundation into your skin, you can keep your makeup in place all day, even in the summer.

Therapy at night

Evening is the time to nurse your tired skin. First, remove all makeup using cotton pads and swabs (see pp. 64–71). Then tone your skin with lotion, nourish it with serum, and finally lock the nutrients in with cream.

Remember to supplement this basic routine with extra care as your skin demands. This includes washing your face with scrub once a week to exfoliate and applying a brightening pack on days when you've spent many hours in the sun.

The attention you give your skin at night will be greatly rewarded the next morning. Going straight to bed without removing your makeup is a big no-no. If this sounds like something you'd do, learn to give your skin more love.

Evening care

1	Cleansing	If you're over 30, use a cream-type cleanser. Lift off any eye makeup and lip color first with makeup remover.
2	Washing	Once you've thoroughly removed your makeup, rinsing with lukewarm water should be sufficient, but if you decide to use facial soap, be sure to lather well.
3	Scrub	Exfoliating your face with scrub every 10 days or so will brighten its color. Mix the scrub with facial soap for a milder texture.
4	Lotion	An ordinary lotion mask (pp. 73–78) will do, but for extra moisture, cover the mask with plastic wrap. This will help your skin better absorb the serum you apply in the next step.
5	Serum	Does your skin need moisture? Is it dry and flaky? Diagnose what it needs and decide which type of serum to use.
6	Emulsion/ cream	Carefully seal in the nutrients you've just fed your skin by spreading on emulsion or cream with the balls of your fingers and palms.

Removing eye and lip makeup

Most of those who have lines and dullness around the eyes or mouth do not cleanse their faces properly. Particular attention is needed for color makeup, such as eye shadow and lipstick, which can cause pigmentation if left unremoved. Always completely wipe these off using makeup remover before moving on to overall cleansing. If you spent 30 minutes putting on makeup, take 30 minutes removing it. This is the mind-set you want to go by.

Also, pearl and shimmer particles tend to be stubborn, so take extra care with removal if you used cosmetics containing them. By properly removing eye and lip makeup first, cleansing your entire face will be much easier.

Preparation

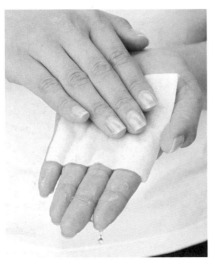 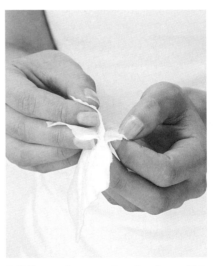

1 Wet a cotton square, then lightly squeeze out the excess moisture between both hands, as shown. Saturate it with a quarter-size amount of makeup remover.

2 Pull apart the cotton into five sheets. This will be easier if you first split one end into five equal parts. Follow the direction in which the fibers run.

Removing eye makeup

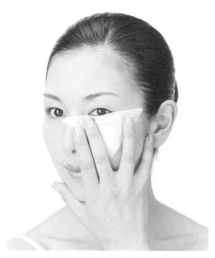

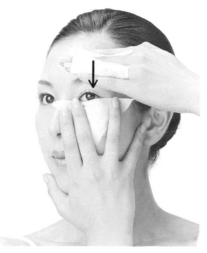

1 Fold the saturated cotton into a triangle and apply it along the lower eyelid.

2 With another sheet held taut between the fingers, transfer the makeup on the upper eyelid onto the first sheet. Use two sheets for each eye.

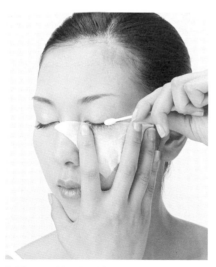

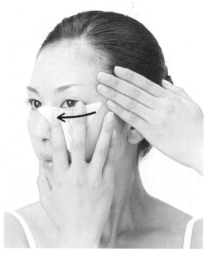

3 Thoroughly take off mascara by transferring it to the lower cotton sheet with a remover-soaked swab. Also remove eyebrow makeup.

4 Finally, with fingers pressed against the temple, slide the cotton inward and off to wipe away residue.

Removing lip makeup

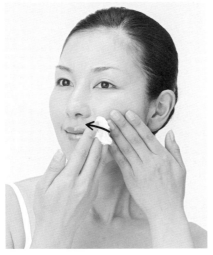

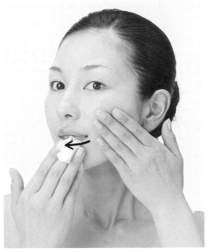

1 With the corners of the mouth firmly lifted, wipe off lip color using the remaining cotton sheet, beginning with the upper lip. On each side of the lip, work inward starting from the corner of your mouth.

2 With the corners still lifted, do the same on the lower lip—one side at a time, working inward. Wipe off carefully, following the contours of the lip.

Cleansing your face

After you've completely removed your eye and lip makeup, it's time for the rest of your face. Note that makeup should first be lifted from the skin before cleansing. Friction is the last thing you want to give your skin, so avoid rubbing off makeup. Instead, lift it off by gently moving your hands in upward and outward movements, with fingers held together to create large surfaces. This will allow you to clear away makeup and dirt down to the pores without stressing the skin.

If you don't know what kind of cleanser to use, I suggest choosing a cream or emulsion type, as they are the least stressful options for the skin.

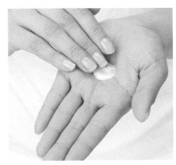

1 Take a nickel-size amount of cleansing cream in your hand and let it warm up.

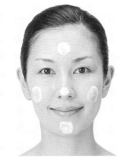

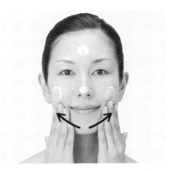

2 Apply it on five spots: both cheeks, the forehead, nose, and chin.

3 Spread the cream from the chin toward the base of the ears. When you get to the ears, press the hollows behind them with your fingertips.

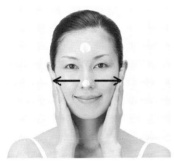

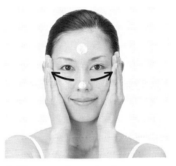

4 Put your hands beside your nose and slide your palms straight outward.

5 Place your fingers by the inner corners of the eyes and spread toward the temples, pulling upward as you do so.

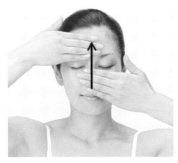

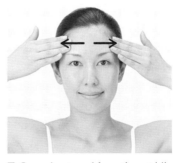

6 Slide alternating hands from the tip of the nose up along the bridge to the forehead.

7 Spread outward from the middle of the forehead.

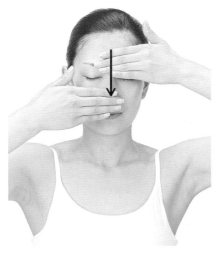

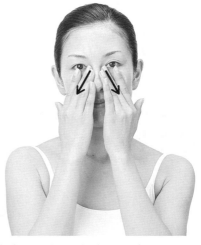

8 Slide alternating hands from the forehead down to the tip of the nose.

9 Gently cleanse both sides of the nose.

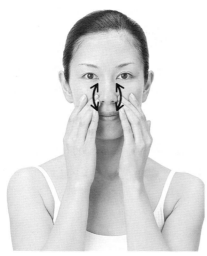

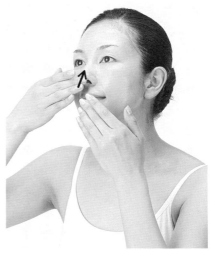

10 Carefully go up and down several times along the wings of the nose with your fingertips.

11 Move your fingers upward around the nostrils.

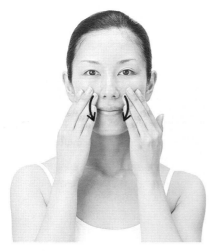

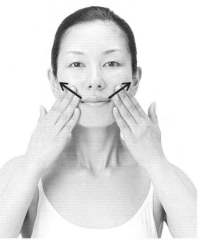

12 Gently press under the nose and spread around the mouth

13 Finally, firmly lift the corners of the mouth.

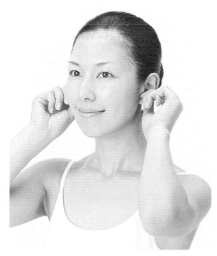

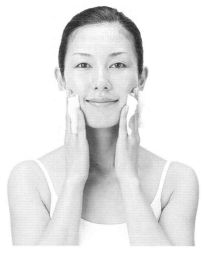

14 Clean the ears, then wipe your hands with tissue.

15 Follow steps 3 to 13 three times. To finish, wipe off your face with wet cotton.

Washing your face and ears

I've observed that many people wash their faces vertically, that is, by moving their hands up and down. This can leave the outer peripheries of the face such as the temples unwashed, and the downward pressure of the hands will gradually lead to sagging. Wash your face with a circular motion from the center outward, imagining that it's a globe.

Rinsing with water should ordinarily be enough. When you wish to use cleansing foam, such as after a sweat, lather it well before use and thoroughly rinse afterward with lukewarm water.

Remember to care for your ears as well after washing your face. Dry and dull ears will make you look older.

Washing your face

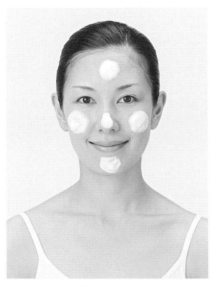 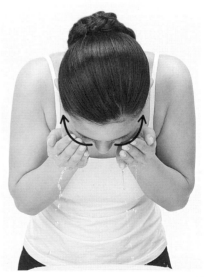

1 Generously lather facial soap or scrub, then apply on the cheeks, forehead, nose, and chin.

2 Wash from the center outward in circles, all the way to the hairline. Be gentle, as rubbing will damage your skin.

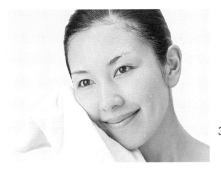

3 To dry, gently press a towel against your skin instead of rubbing up and down. Think of absorbing the moisture.

Washing your ears

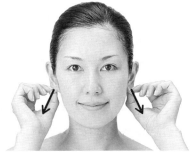

1 Your ears are also part of your face; they, too, should be washed and massaged. First, pull the earlobes downward.

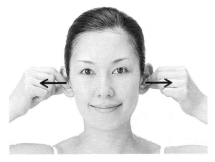

2 Next, hold the middle of your ears and pull sideways. There are pressure points all over the ears.

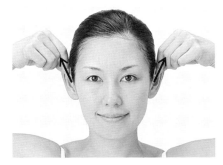

3 Hold the top of your ears and pull diagonally upward. This routine will improve your complexion.

Exfoliating with facial scrub

It's best to exfoliate the skin with facial scrub at least once a week. The fine particles of scrub will whisk away dead cells and dirt, giving your skin greater clarity. Also, your skin will better absorb lotions and other cosmetics. If you feel the grains to be too abrasive, try mixing the scrub with the same amount of facial soap and further smoothing it out with lukewarm water.

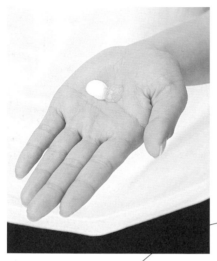

For a milder texture, mix equal parts scrub and facial soap and add a few drops of lukewarm water, then lather well. Wash gently so as to whisk away dead cells.

The three-minute lotion mask

If you spritz water on a piece of paper, the water will sit on the surface of the paper, then gradually evaporate, leaving the paper parched and puckered. But if you place a damp towel on the paper and let it sit there for a bit, the paper will gradually absorb the water and become moist.

The same principle applies to your surface skin, which is said to be about a hundredth of an inch thick. To get your skin to absorb the active ingredients in a lotion, allow the lotion to sink into it by using a damp cotton pad. This is far more beneficial than simply spraying or dabbing lotion on your face.

The greatest thing about the lotion mask I introduce here is its simplicity. It's as easy as wetting a cotton pad with water, pouring a quarter-size amount of lotion on it, and putting it on your face for three minutes. Cotton, water, lotion, and three minutes of your time are all you need.

Nonquilted absorbent cotton pads work best. The ones I use— my own brand, currently available only in Japan—are about 3 inches by 6 inches, with a thickness of about a fifth of an inch, but you can use whatever size is available. (A lotion mask technique that uses cotton widely available in the U.S. and elsewhere follows the method I introduce here.) I cut the cotton in half, and then after dampening the squares with water and lotion, which helps control the "fuzz factor," I pull them apart into thin layers before applying them to my face.

This homemade mask will save you money, because you don't need to use as much lotion as you would with dry cotton or spray bottles. Suspending the lotion on damp cotton won't dilute your lotion's effectiveness either, but merely spread it further and allow it to sink in.

By soothing and hydrating your skin with a lotion mask, you can refine its texture and instantly make it supple. That's why I say lotion masks are as effective as serums.

Chizu Saeki's original lotion mask

For this technique, you need to use thick (0.2 inch) cotton squares that can be pulled apart into layers.

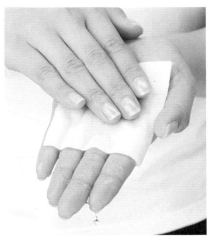

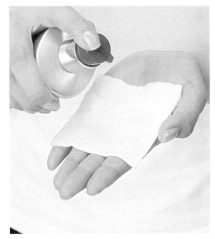

1 Wet a cotton pad with water and lightly squeeze.

2 Saturate the pad with a quarter-size amount of lotion.

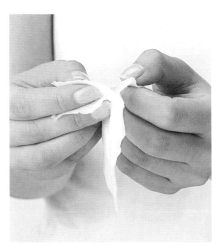

3 Pull the pad apart into five thin layers. It should be easier to split the layers in the direction that the fibers run.

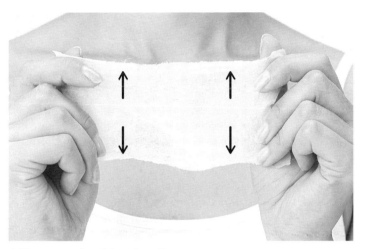

4 You can stretch each layer by pulling it gently side to side before placing it on your face.

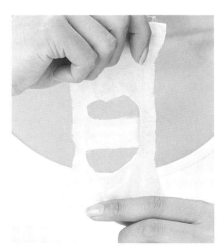

5 Open up holes in one of the layers for the nose and mouth.

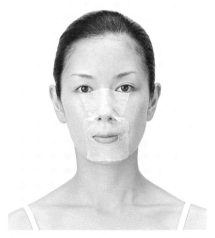

6 Cover the lower half of your face, from under the eyes to the chin, using the piece of cotton with the holes cut out.

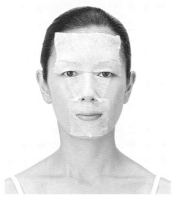

7 Cover your forehead with another piece of cotton.

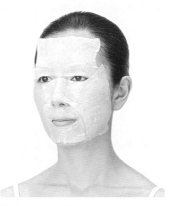

8 Cover your left cheek.

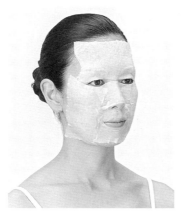

9 Cover your right cheek.

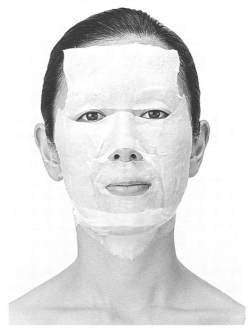

10 Cover your chin and neck with the remaining piece, and let sit for three minutes. Don't keep the mask on any longer than three minutes, or the moisture will begin to evaporate.

The international lotion mask

This lotion mask uses Miss Webril 100% Cotton Skin Care Pads, available in the U.S. and elsewhere.

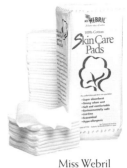

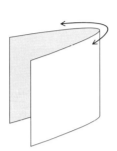 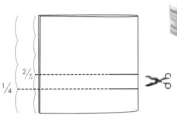

Miss Webril
100% Cotton
Skin Care Pads

1 Take one 8 × 4 inch cotton pad and fold it in half. Cut out breathing holes for the nose and mouth roughly two-fifths and one-fourth of the way along the folded edge, depending on the distance between your nose and mouth.

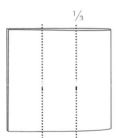 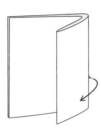 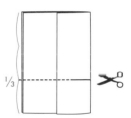

2 Fold another piece of cotton in half, and then fold again in thirds. Cut out holes for the eyes about one-third of the way along the folded edge.

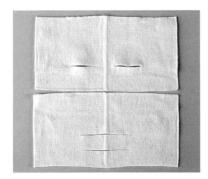

The cotton should look like this.

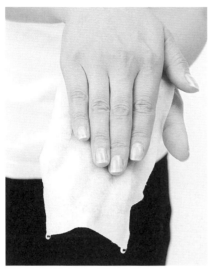

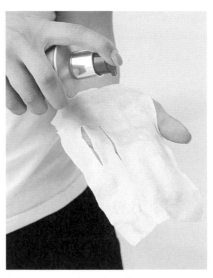

3 Wet both pads with water and lightly squeeze.

4 Saturate each pad with a quarter-size amount of lotion.

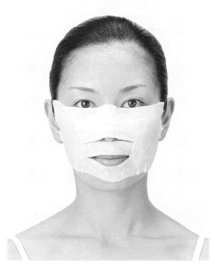

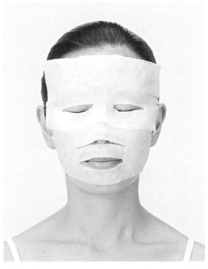

5 Apply the nose-and-mouth piece across the lower half of your face.

6 Apply the eyes piece across the upper half of your face. Let the mask sit on your face for three minutes. Don't keep the mask on any longer than three minutes, or the moisture will begin to evaporate.

Applying serum

After conditioning the skin surface with lotion, next comes serum. Serums are supplements to nourish your skin; they reach deep into the dermal layer—responsible for firmness and elasticity—to give your skin fullness and vigor. I strongly encourage those over the age of 25 to use serum morning and evening.

The basic steps are to warm the serum in your hands, then dab it on five spots on your face and spread it in upward and outward motions. By moving your hands in the shape of the letter V, you can give your face a lift at the same time. You should follow the product directions regarding the amount, but roughly two to three pumps' worth should be about right. If this isn't enough, add another pump.

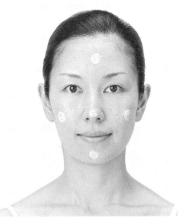

1 After warming the serum in your hands, apply it on both cheeks, your forehead, nose, and chin.

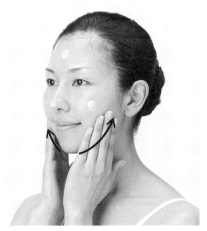

2 Spread the serum on the chin toward the base of the ears. With the flats of your fingers, pull up the muscles around your chin and mouth while forming a V with the hands.

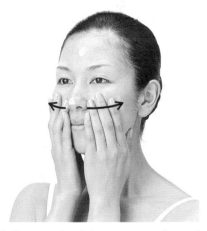

3 Place your hands by your nose and spread straight out toward your ears.

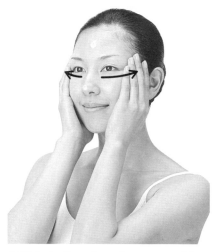

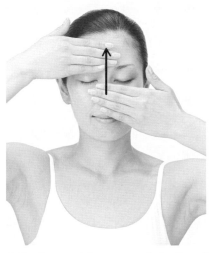

4 With the flats of your fingers, spread from the inner corners of the eyes to the temples while gently pulling the muscles upward.

5 Gently spread the serum with the flats of your fingers, sliding alternating hands from the tip of the nose up along the bridge.

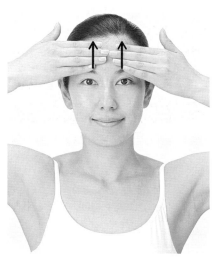

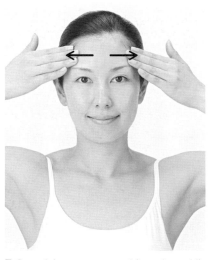

6 Further spread upward from between the eyebrows toward the middle of the forehead, again pulling up the muscles.

7 Spread the serum outward from the middle of the forehead with the flats of your fingers, stretching the muscles as well.

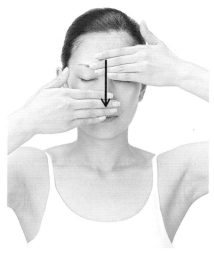

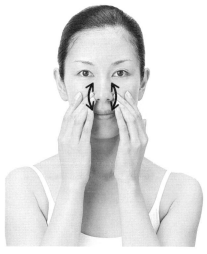

8 Bring your fingers back to the middle and slide alternating hands from the forehead down to the tip of the nose.

9 Don't forget the wings of the nose. Lightly go up and down both sides with your fingertips.

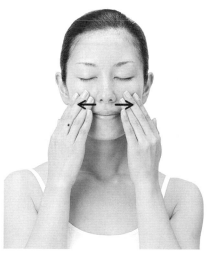

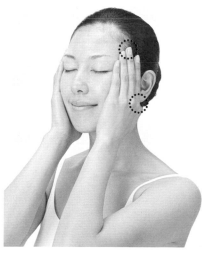

10 From under the nose, spread the serum so as to gently stretch the muscles toward the corners of the mouth.

11 Let the serum's nutrients reach deep into the skin by gently pressing your face with both hands, with the middle fingers on the temples and the thumbs in the hollows behind the ears.

Prevent skin aging with daily sun protection

You may or may not be aware that the sun's ultraviolet rays not only tan your skin but can cause it to wrinkle and sag. They penetrate through the depths of your skin and ruin the inner tissue. Rather than wait until after you've been exposed and the damage has been done, it's better to take preventive care. In Australia, where UV radiation is strong, thorough sun protection is recommended even for children, given the risk of skin cancer.

Meanwhile, it's also true that a lot of sunscreen lotions are not comfortable to use, or contain ingredients that aren't good for the skin. Some people may also find it a hassle to have to apply yet another product on their faces.

Here's what I do: after my morning skincare regimen, I blend equal parts sunscreen and either emulsion or primer and apply the mixture on my face. This reduces the stickiness of the sunscreen, helping it to spread easily and smoothly. The moisturizing effect of the emulsion or primer will give your skin luster, and if you use a tinted type, you can even conceal any dullness in your skin. On days that I don't wear foundation, I use this technique to kill three birds with one stone—light makeup, sun protection, and moisturizing. It also saves time, since you only need to apply one coating.

CHAPTER 5

Cures for Problem Skin

When I turned 40, my skin went through hell. But by looking after it carefully day after day, I was able to solve most of the major problems.

Preventing and repairing skin problems

You can put on the most fabulous dress, but if you're not in shape, it will look as if the dress is wearing you, not you wearing the dress. I like describing surface skincare in terms of clothing. No amount of deluxe cream will make you look truly beautiful if your underlying dermis and the muscles that animate and define your face have been neglected. Although surface skin tends to be the focus of facial routines, I'd like you to strive for beauty in more holistic terms.

The foods you eat, the supplements you take, your cosmetics and serums should all be part of the program. For example, suppose your face appears to be less firm than usual. In this case, it's particularly important to pay attention to both your skin and the underlying muscles. If your face is losing firmness, it isn't happening just on the top layer. The skin sags because the muscles underneath lose the strength to keep it in place. So applying skincare products isn't enough to cope with the problem; you need to exercise the underlying muscles to prevent sagging and wrinkles while treating your skin to repair any damage you might already have.

Adopting a holistic approach, one that goes beyond the superficial layer targeted by most cosmetics, will dramatically improve your skin condition.

Troubleshooting: the basic tactics

Improvements from within: diet and supplements

I make a point of consuming mineral water, vegetables, and fruits every day. Vitamins C and E and calcium are especially important for skin beauty. Make sure you're taking enough of these nutrients, using the help of dietary supplements if need be.

Caring for the epidermis: cosmetics and massage

Epidermal care includes cleansing to remove dirt, lotion masks to refine the surface, and exfoliation of dead cells. This sequence is effective for breakouts and dullness, since it softens your skin and keeps it clean.

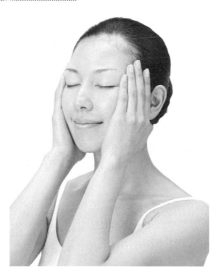

Nourishing the dermis: serum

The skin sags and brown spots darken when the dermis isn't fully functioning. Use serum to repair the dermis. Different serums serve different purposes: brightening serum helps erase brown spots, collagen- and elastin-enriched serum fights sagging, and so forth.

Toning the muscles: exercises and massage

Muscles will waste away if they're in disuse. The skin around the eyes and cheeks sags easily, and wrinkles tend to form as well. Make sure to work out the muscles in addition to caring for the skin.

Wrinkles

Wrinkles are caused by the skin's ingrained habit patterns. The first step in caring for wrinkled skin is to "loosen" those habits by coaxing the skin in the opposite direction. Forehead wrinkles usually form horizontally, for instance, so they should be eased by pinching them vertically, or from the sides. The laugh lines that form vertically on both sides of the mouth, meanwhile, should be pinched horizontally—from above and below. The idea is to "reset" the skin's habits by pinching the lines perpendicularly to the direction in which they run.

To treat crow's feet and fine lines around the eyes, smooth out the wrinkles with the fingers while tapping eye cream onto the skin. Be creative with how you smooth out different kinds of wrinkles: if you have lines extending outward from the outer corners of the eyes, for instance, you may want to smooth them inward.

Deep lines will take longer to treat, so take early action.

1 Fine wrinkles

2 Crow's feet

3 Deep creases in the forehead, between the brows, and around the mouth

1 Fine wrinkles

The skin around the eyes is prone to fine wrinkles resembling the crinkled texture of crepe fabric. The wrinkles run in many directions, so smooth out vertical wrinkles horizontally and horizontal wrinkles vertically with one hand as you carefully rub in eye cream or eye serum with the fingertips of the other hand.

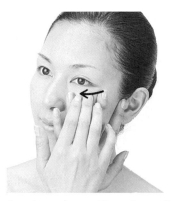

Stretch out the wrinkles and nourish them with eye cream.

2 Crow's feet

Wrinkles at the corners of the eyes, called crow's feet, form when the skin lacks moisture and oil. Feed your skin both: moisture in the morning with eye serum, and oil at night with eye cream. The skin around the eyes is delicate, so slide your fingers from the outer edge inward while holding the skin in place with the other hand.

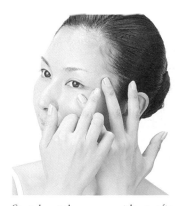

Stretch out the creases with your fingers and apply serum or cream with light taps of the other middle finger.

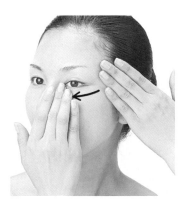

Hold down the corner of your eye and rub in the cosmetic from the outside inward with the middle and ring fingers of the other hand.

3 Deep creases in the forehead, between the brows, and around the mouth

Deep creases in the forehead, between the brows, and around the mouth give you a tired impression. Start by easing the skin out of the shape it has hardened into. By doing these loosening massages, you'll not only erase wrinkles over time, but also get more mileage out of your cosmetics.

Deep creases in the forehead

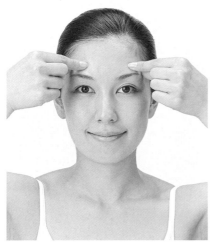

Pinch the horizontal forehead lines from both sides.

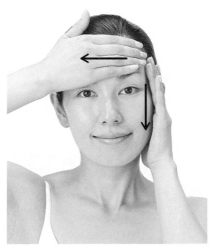

Stretch the skin sideways along the creases.

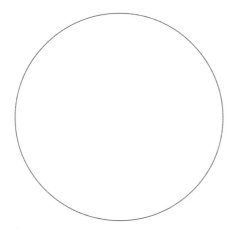

Deep creases between the brows

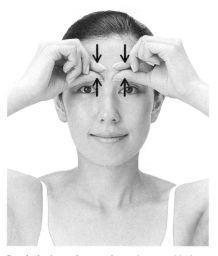

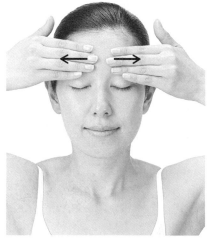

Pinch the brow furrows from above and below.

Pull outward so as to erase the vertical lines.

Deep creases around the mouth

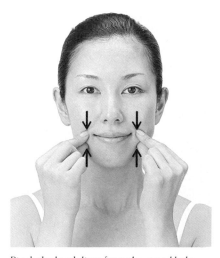

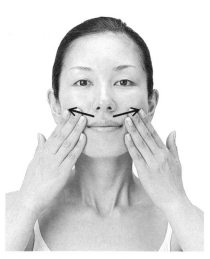

Pinch the laugh lines from above and below.

Pull outward so as to erase the vertical lines.

Sagging

Those who spend long hours looking down doing office work, who don't talk with other people often, or whose left and right sides are poorly balanced should beware of facial sagging and double chins.

Sagging happens because the muscles supporting the skin grow weak, and you can't repair it by caring for surface skin alone. You need to use other remedies—massages to improve lymph flow, packs to firm up the face, and, most of all, muscular exercises to tone the facial muscles.

I've made a habit of lifting my cheeks whenever it occurs to me. You may think this simple action wouldn't amount to much, but you can actually prevent sagging with little efforts like this.

As for the neck, which is prone to horizontal lines caused by sagging skin, I suggest massaging it with neck cream.

1 Sagging neck

2 Sagging cheeks

3 Sagging mouth

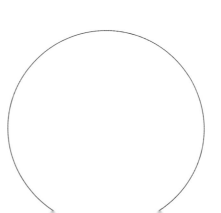

1 Sagging neck

Take plenty of neck cream in your hands and press the hollows behind the earlobes, where lymph nodes are located. Then massage your neck with alternating hands, gripping the left side with your right hand and the right side with your left. Think of draining the lymphatic waste toward the collarbones.

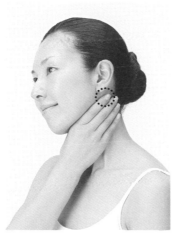

1 Grip your neck and press the lymph nodes in the hollow behind your ear

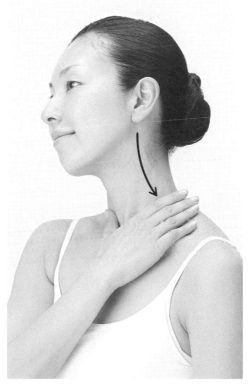

2 Drain the lymphatic waste toward the collarbone.

2 Sagging cheeks

Remedy sagging cheeks in three steps. Once a day, hold your cheeks in your hands and slowly lift them 10 times. Next, firm your face with a pack; this will give you quick results. Last, try an oral exercise. Work out your underused cheek muscles by pronouncing the five Japanese vowels, which are quite similar to English a, e, i, o, u.

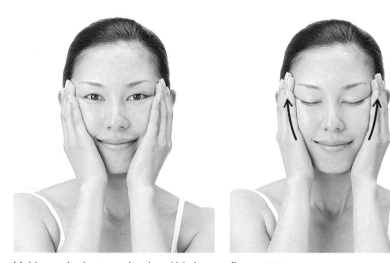

Hold your cheeks in your hands and lift them up. Repeat 10 times.

For the oral exercise, open your mouth wide and slowly voice the vowels: "ah-ay-ee-oh-oo." This exercise helps counter sagging and distortion by activating the muscles of your entire face. For those who spend long hours working at a desk or don't often talk with others, I recommend doing this exercise whenever and as many times as you like.

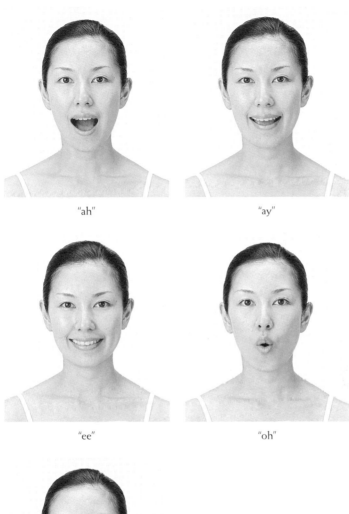

"ah"

"ay"

"ee"

"oh"

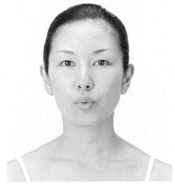

"oo"

3 Sagging mouth

For sagging in the corners of the mouth, lift the sides of your lips by pinching them with your thumbs and forefingers. For vertical lines above the lips, ease the area with three fingers together. Finally, form a clown smile to see which side gets furrowed deeper and droops more at the corner. Make a conscious effort to chew food on that side.

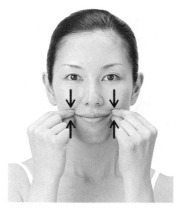

Pinch and lift the corners of the mouth.

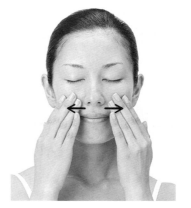

Press and smooth the vertical lines above the lips outward with your fingers.

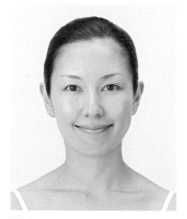

Widen your mouth into a big clown smile with lips closed to check for sagging.

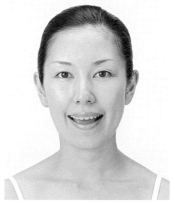

Tone the muscles around your mouth with vowel exercises (previous page).

Oily skin

There are many possible causes of oily skin, such as too much oily food in one's diet, too much face washing, or too much oil cleansing. But one characteristic shared by people with oily skin is that they are bent on removing the oil.

If this sounds like you, here's a word of advice: don't try to remove the oil, as it will only give your skin the message that it's deficient in oil and needs to produce more. What you should be thinking about is achieving an oil and moisture balance. The skin produces too much oil when it's dry, so if your skin is oily, think of supplying it with moisture.

Meanwhile, if you're greasy in the T-zone but peeling at the tip of your nose, you'll need to tweak the basic skincare techniques to fit your circumstances, such as by putting a lotion mask on just the dry parts of your face.

1 Oily T-zone
2 Greasy face

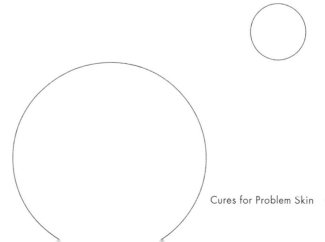

1 Oily T-zone

It's natural for the forehead, nose, and chin to produce oil. But if you feel your T-zone is too greasy, you can improve the moisture and oil balance by putting a lotion mask on just that part of your face, or at least on the nose. If the rest of your face is fine, partial treatment will do: apply a brightening pack on the T-zone or scrub-wash only persistently oily areas.

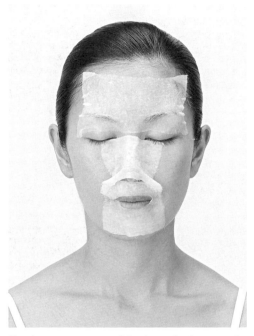

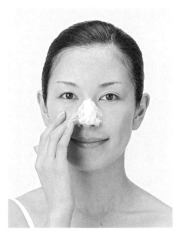

Exfoliate dead skin cells by washing with scrub.

Condition greasy parts of the skin with a lotion mask.

2 Greasy face

Washing your face with soap after using makeup remover robs your skin of vital moisture and only makes it oilier. Supply moisture to counter greasiness. Hydrate your skin from inside by drinking plenty of water and from outside by applying lotion masks. You'll find your skin stops producing excessive oil and plumps out, making the pores less noticeable.

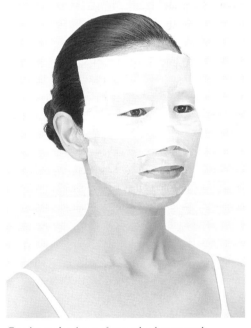

Condition the skin surface with a lotion mask.

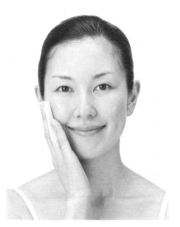

To take away excessive oil, press dampened cotton against your face rather than using blotting paper.

Pimples and breakouts

The oil secreted from sebaceous glands and moisture secreted by sweat glands blend together on the skin surface. The result is a natural cream that protects our skin. But when the skin overproduces oil or is covered with a layer of dead cells, the oil will clog the glands, causing inflammation or infection. This is how pimples and breakouts form.

Unlike adolescent acne, which breaks out all at once and ebbs just as quickly, adult pimples are stubborn and recur in the same spots. Popping pimples with your fingernails can cause scars and pigmentation, so you need to treat them with care. The same goes for premenstrual acne. Rather than trying to remove pimples on the spot, think of flushing them out from the inside by improving your skin's metabolism.

If your skin is prone to premenstrual breakouts, take preventive action, such as improving bodily circulation with lymph massages and conditioning the skin surface by exfoliating. Pimples and breakouts that have already formed, meanwhile, should be treated by careful removal of the core, followed by a brightening pack to prevent pigmentation.

Of course, the best way to deal with pimples is to not get them. Lack of sleep, too much stress, and poor cleansing, as well as overeating and overdrinking, all lead to pimples and breakouts. Simply avoid these, and you should see a notable difference in your skin condition.

1 Adult acne

2 Premenstrual acne

1 Adult acne

If you find a pimple that you just cannot leave alone, try following these steps. Soak a piece of cotton with a lotion containing alcohol and disinfect just the pimple and surrounding area. If the pimple has a core, loosen it by jiggling and pinching the skin around it. Then, to prevent pigmentation, put on a brightening pack. Also remember to exfoliate weekly with facial scrub.

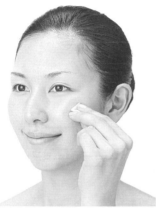

1 Disinfect the affected area with alcohol-soaked cotton.

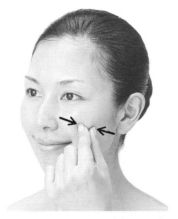

2 Jiggle the skin around the pimple with your fingertips.

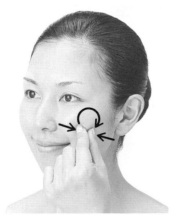

3 Moving in a circle around the pimple, gently pinch the surrounding skin so as to loosen the core.

2 Premenstrual acne

A woman's metabolism rate falls right before her period, making her skin susceptible to clogged pores and pimples. It's therefore important to act early by exfoliating and clearing pores with facial scrub and brightening packs. It also helps to loosen stiffened skin and drain out waste matter with lymph massages.

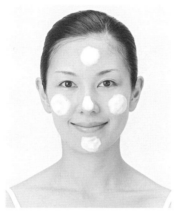
Exfoliate dead skin cells with scrub.

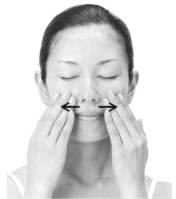
Massage acne-prone areas.

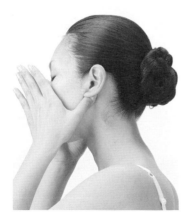
Drain out waste matter with lymph massages (pp. 54–59).

Clogged pores and blackheads

If you have a habit of unclogging pores by pushing out the dirt with your fingers, stop immediately. This ruins your skin, and doing it repeatedly will only further enlarge your pores. And even if you feel better because you've gotten rid of the dirt, the skin will redden and harden, causing the pores to stand out more than ever.

Pores are holes, so the key to making them stand out less is to plump out the skin around them. Do this by moisturizing your skin with a lotion mask. If you're doing a lotion mask on your entire face, there's no need to separately treat your nose.

The next step is to tighten the pores by cooling down the skin with plastic-wrapped ice cubes. Slowly move the ice along the muscles of your face, adding gentle pressure.

This lotion pack and cooling routine should be done every day.

For blackheads, wash your face with a facial soap containing scrub grains about once a week.

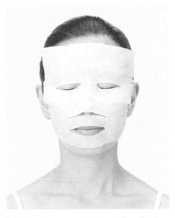

Moisturize your skin with a lotion mask (pp. 73–78).

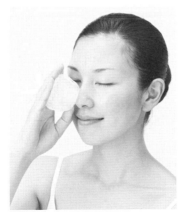

Cool down the skin around the troubled area with an ice cube wrapped in plastic wrap. Push the cube gently along your muscles.

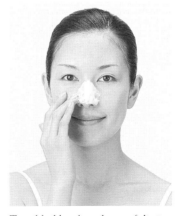

Treat blackheads with an exfoliating facial soap. Scrub in circles, gently.

BEAUTY COLUMN

Color your world

Color greatly affects a woman's beauty. Pink is said to show off a woman's beauty best, so the towels, gowns, and other effects at my salon are all a soft pink.

People who are busy with home or office duties often don't realize how "gray" they have become in both mind and body. Incorporate your favorite color in your home decor and give your spirit a lift. Once your mind is refreshed, your skin is sure to come back to life as well.

In addition to color, another potent remedy is fragrance. We've all seen the blissful expression someone gets breathing in the sweet fragrance of flowers. The magic that fragrances offer us shows up as beauty on our faces. Nowadays, you can find a wide range of aromatherapy items for the home, or to carry around with you, to give your day a whiff of pleasure.

Our brains generate alpha waves when we're in a state of relaxation or euphoria. These brain waves are beneficial for our emotional and physical health—and for our skin—because they enhance our natural healing power. When we're tensed up or stressed, meanwhile, our healing power declines, making us more prone to disease and skin problems.

Living in a busy world, we're likely to end the day without having generated any alpha waves. Make an effort to find time in your everyday life to free your mind and body by offering them a moment of pleasure.

CHAPTER 6

Quick Fix
Spa Secrets

Meeting a friend you haven't seen for ages? Got a hot date? Have an important interview tomorrow? No worries—here are some emergency remedies for quick results.

Instant steam pack with a shower cap

Back in my days working for a cosmetics company, when I used to travel a lot on business, one problem that always plagued me was the dryness of hotel rooms. I needed to find some way of dealing with it; I couldn't possibly receive clients with flaky dry skin.

The emergency treatment I came up with was to cut holes into a shower cap that happened to be in the bathroom and wear it over my face after the usual skincare. Surprisingly enough, my skin instantly went from parched to moist and succulent.

Here I will share with you the quick and easy steam pack that I invented. There are only three steps, actually: cut one or two holes in a shower cap, apply a lotion mask (pp. 73–78), and then cover your face with the cap. In two to three minutes, your body heat combined with the lotion's moisture will turn the inside of the shower cap into a steam sauna.

Since little evaporation occurs, unlike with a lotion mask alone, the shower cap can be left on for five or ten minutes. The moisture will deeply penetrate your skin, giving it clarity.

Steam pack

If you do this while sitting in the bath, even if you're just wearing a shower cap over your face without a lotion mask, it will do wonders.

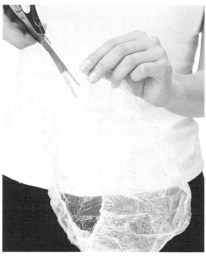

1 Cut two slits into a shower cap for breathing.

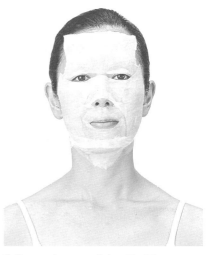

2 Put on a lotion mask (pp. 73–78).

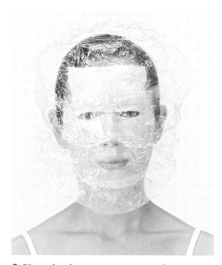

3 Place the shower cap over your face.

Warm care for unwinding your mind and body

For days when . . .

- You've been out shopping in the wind and cold
- You've been stuck in an overly air-conditioned room
- You've numbed your skin skiing or playing in the snow
- You're having your period and you feel chilled
- You're stressed out

The sight of cats napping in the sun by a window brings smiles to our faces. Cats instinctively know the coziest spots in the house. As for us, on wintry days, we enjoy relaxing with a cup of coffee in a café or curling up by a toasty fire.

The skin is just the same: on chilly days, it wants warmth too. When our skin is cold, the pores squeeze shut and won't let cosmetics through. On days like this, it's necessary to "defrost" your skin—make it warm—before getting on with your skincare routine.

The best way to warm up your skin is to take a nice, long bath. But if you're short on time, you can simply spread a hot towel over your face. If you've ever experienced a hot towel wrap at a hair salon or spa, you'll know just how relaxing these warming treatments can be.

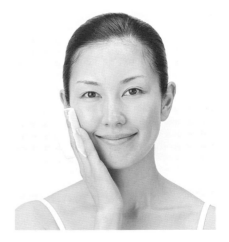

1 Cleansing

Cleanse your entire face after removing mascara, eye color, and lipstick (pp. 64–69). Use cotton squares to remove the overall makeup, and cotton swabs around the eyes.

2 Hot towel

Soak a towel with hot water, wring it gently, then microwave it for 30 seconds in plastic wrap. Remove the plastic wrap and spread the towel over your face and ears to open tightened pores and make your skin more receptive to care.

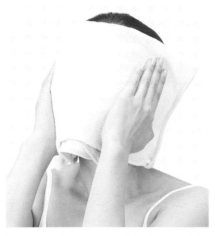 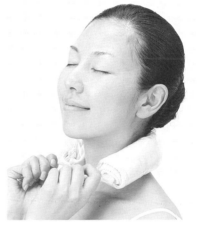

Cover your face and ears with a hot towel for three minutes.

Place a rolled-up hot towel, wrapped in plastic wrap, under your neck. it's very relaxing.

3 Lotion

Once you've revived your icy skin, give it a lotion mask (pp. 73–78).

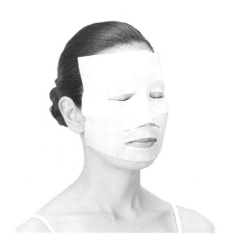

4 Massage

Massage your entire face, gently pressing the tense muscles with your fingers. If you want to use massage cream,
choose one that soothes or moistur-
izes. Blood and lymph flow will be
stimulated as you loosen the muscles,
giving your face a healthier color.

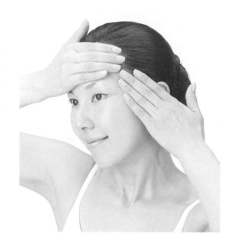

5 Serum

Now that you've conditioned your surface skin, it's time to send
nourishing serum into the dermis. You can apply two different
kinds—like a rejuvenating serum plus a moisturizer—when your
skin is extra tired.

6 Cream

Top everything off with cream to seal in the moisture and nutrients. Rather than an emulsion, go for a cream, the more moisturizing of the two, when your skin has had a cold and dry day. The
best is one that firms and elasticizes.

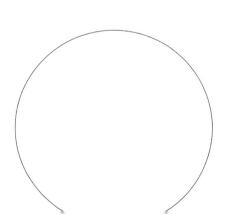

Cool care for soothing your body and skin

For days when . . .

- You've been in the heat and sun for hours
- You've played sports or looked after your kids all morning
- Your skin is flushed from running errands
- Something has upset you
- Your skin has gone clammy because of the humidity

Athletes often cool inflamed areas with an ice spray or cold pack. The lotion mask I suggest is a bit like a cold pack in that it soothes and tones your overheated or irritated skin, making way for other skincare products to seep in.

In addition to including lotion masks in your daily routine, I recommend the cool-down treatment outlined on the following pages. All you need are a refrigerated wet towel, a spray bottle (you can pick one up at a dollar store, or recycle one), and ice. Although simply utilizing familiar items you're likely to have at home, this is actually a professional-quality treatment that I offer at my salon. Use this technique whenever you want to restore your skin to its normal condition and temperature.

1 Cleansing

Cleanse your entire face after removing mascara, eye color, and lipstick (pp. 64–69). Use cotton squares to remove the overall make-up, and cotton swabs around the eyes.

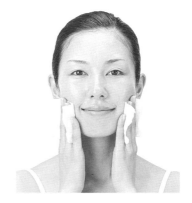

2 Cold towel

During the hot season, keep a few towels wrapped in plastic in your refrigerator. Place one of these towels over your face to relieve the heat. Also, doing this in the morning after washing your face will tighten your pores and help your makeup stay in place.

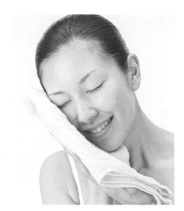

Cover your face and ears with a cold towel.

3 Water spray

A handy way of further calming your skin is a water massage (pp.112–13). Simply spray your face using a spray bottle or plastic wash bottle; something from a dollar shop or discount store will do. Directly watering the skin will instantly rehydrate it.

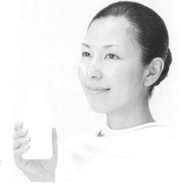

Spray your face with a jet of water along the muscles.

4 Ice

The quickest remedy for cooling down overheated skin is ice. Cold packs are also recommended.

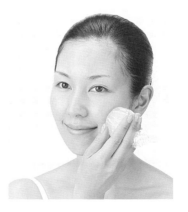

Roll plastic-wrapped ice along your face.

5 Lotion

Apply a lotion mask (pp. 73–78). Spread a shower cap (with breathing holes cut out) over this for extra effect.

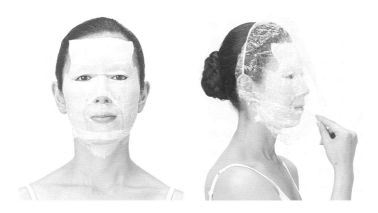

6 Pack

When you have blackheads from sweating or encountering dirt, apply a brightening pack at night. If washing your face is the equivalent of doing your laundry at home, using a pack is like going to a professional cleaner's. By morning you'll see great results—fresh and remarkably clean.

7 Serum

Use a brightening serum on dull skin and a moisturizing type on dehydrated skin. Also use eye treatment if you're feeling dry around the eyes. Be sure to rub the serum into your laugh lines and fine wrinkles, if you have any.

8 Cream

After checking your skin's condition and amply nourishing it accordingly, seal it with cream or emulsion. Choose cream for a stronger barrier, particularly if you're over 30.

Water massage to energize your skin

People who exercise by working out their various muscles can stay in shape for a good many years. In the same way, you can keep your face from sagging by regularly exercising your facial muscles. But I advise against facial training that makes you strain your muscles to form unnatural expressions; it's unpleasant, and can also cause wrinkles.

The ideal way to tone your facial muscles is to activate them while putting minimum stress on your skin. I recommend a special water massage, which will invigorate your facial muscles without stressing your surface skin.

To perform a water massage, prepare a "swan-neck," or wash bottle of the sort you can buy online (see p. 26). Fill the bottle with purified or distilled water, available for a small sum at drugstores and supermarkets.

All you need to do is spray the water evenly over your face, following the muscle structure. A bit of force is needed to get a massaging effect, so spray the water from a short distance with just enough pressure to feel the stimulation.

I offer this treatment at my salon. It instantly energizes the skin, and it's also good for those who have problems with enlarged pores. Massaging your face with water will rehydrate and plump out your skin and minimize your pores.

Water massage

The key is to spray water along the muscles of facial expression. The basic direction of the massage is consistently an inward and upward motion. Spray in the following order and repeat: the forehead, around the right eye, the right cheek, around the mouth, the left cheek, around the left eye, down the nose, and then once around the entire face.

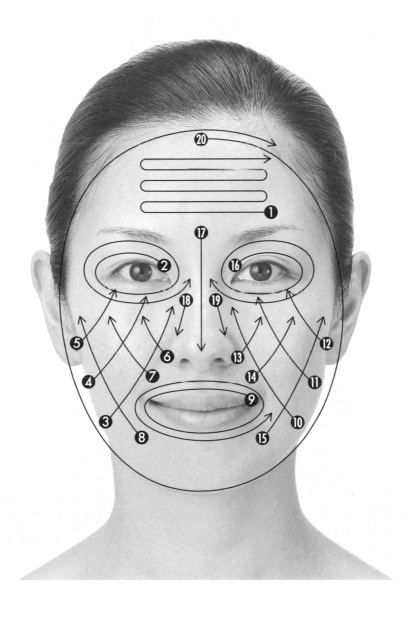

Moist lips with honey and lymph massage

Your lips can get chapped for a variety of reasons. If your stomach is troubled from excessive eating and drinking, if you have a vitamin E deficiency, if you've eaten too much spicy food, or even if you've just been in the sun or dry weather for too long, your lips could suffer. When your lips are cracked or peeling, even lipstick and gloss can't make them look better.

I suggest using honey at times like this. Applying honey on chapped lips is an age-old remedy, and there are many lip-care products containing honey. Honey is a natural moisturizer, and it's also safe to lick and is known for its benefits as a health food.

Keep a jar of honey handy in your kitchen so you can give your lips a honey pack whenever they feel dry. All it takes is to put plenty of honey on your lips and cover them with a piece of plastic wrap cut to size. Your lips will become moist in a matter of five minutes.

Along with the honey pack, I advise you to do lymph massages for your lips. This involves massaging your jawline with the balls of your thumbs, slowly proceeding from the chin to the back of the ears. Focus on the lymph flow as you do so. If your lips are looking dull, this will give them a pinkish glow.

I do this massage every morning before putting on lip color. The natural rosy color of your lips will enhance the color of your lipstick.

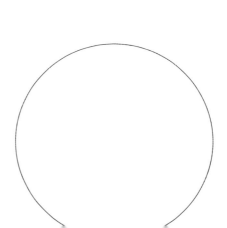

Honey pack

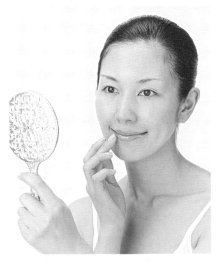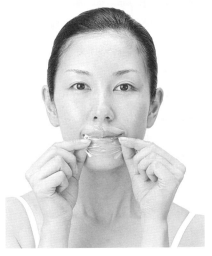

1 Put plenty of honey on your lips.

2 Cover your lips with plastic wrap.

Lymph massage

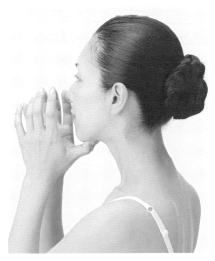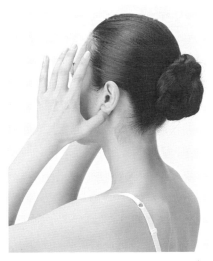

1 With the balls of your thumbs, press the lymph nodes that run from underneath your chin toward your ears.

2 Drain out waste matter by pressing on the lymph nodes behind the ears.

Chizu's golden formula: look ten years younger in one night

If you're anticipating a special day—a friend's wedding, a date, a school reunion—you'll want your skin in great shape, and that means getting started from the evening before. It'll be too late to sit in front of the mirror on the day of the event and despair at how horrible your skin looks. You can give yourself salon-quality treatment and have luminous skin with a bit of forethought and effort. Here's the regimen I suggest.

1 The night before your event, put on a lotion mask (pp. 73–78) to condition your skin.

2 Further moisturize your skin with vapor by using a shower cap or a sheet of plastic wrap (with breathing holes cut out) to seal the mask.

3 To get the most out of this treatment, do the above while sitting in the bath.

4 Remove the mask and massage your face with massage cream to restore your skin's firmness, luster, and elasticity. Focus on the lymph flow as you do so and push out waste matter to relieve swelling.

5 Cover your face with a steam towel for five minutes. It's time to take off the towel when it gets cold. This will open your pores, readying your skin for the moisture and nutrients to follow. To prepare a steam towel, simply soak a towel with hot water, wring it out, then microwave it for about 30 seconds. Be careful not to burn yourself!

6 Energize your skin with a water massage (pp. 112–13).

7 Apply serum, rubbing it in so as to deliver it into the deeper layers.

8 Seal your skin with cream, rather than emulsion, to help it retain the moisture and nutrients you've sent into the deeper layers.

9 Before applying makeup the next morning, tighten the pores by placing a cold towel against your face. Your makeup will go on more smoothly and won't need to be fixed all day.

Morning special: worn-out skin rescue

We all have those mornings when our skin condition is so bad it's depressing to look in the mirror— when we're stressed out, didn't get enough sleep, a period is coming up, or we were out all night. It's hard to get in the mood to leave the house on days like this. But here are some tricks you can use to quickly revive your skin, and your spirit.

1 Put on a lotion mask (pp. 73–78) to condition your skin.

2 Cover your face with a cold towel to tighten your pores. A towel that's been soaked with water and wrung out is fine, but better yet, keep two or three damp hand towels in the refrigerator so you can grab one whenever you need it.

3 Apply a brightening or firming pack for three minutes. Though people tend to think of evening as the best time for packs, morning is also good, since packs provide immediate results. You'll find your skin looking lighter than before.

4 Apply plenty of serum.

5 Seal your skin with treatment cream.

6 Put on foundation primer.

7 Choose liquid foundation with a moist finish rather than a matte finish. When your skin isn't in good condition, always use liquid foundation and not a powder type; it'll adhere to your skin better. Apply the foundation with your fingers as if you're trying to push the particles into your pores. This will simultaneously help keep your makeup from coming off and provide a light massage to improve your blood circulation.

Take beauty into your own hands

Today, we're bombarded with a multitude of signs advertising cosmetics, facial treatments, and spa & beauty salons. From experience, I know it's hard to find products or salons that give you good value for your money. You might casually walk into a department store or salon, only to end up paying an absurd amount of money because you were talked into buying the products or treatments sold there.

You'll be much better off learning how to make yourself beautiful with your own hands. After all, if you stop and think about it, no one—not even the most experienced esthetician—knows your skin as well as you do. You, of all people, have the greatest potential to become your best esthetician. And, once you learn how to achieve your best skin naturally, you'll find that many expensive cosmetics or treatments are simply unnecessary.

There's no need to pay for professional services or costly products if you're treating yourself at home. By practicing the methods in this book while listening to your favorite music—or even better, while sitting in the bath—you'll feel your mind and body being liberated. What better quality time could you ask for?

Be your own esthetician from today. Your skin will respond to the love you give it with visible results.

Diagnosing Your Skin Type

How well do you know your skin? Skin types vary from one person to the next, just as our personalities and faces differ. The first step to achieving perfect skin is to get to know your skin type. Here are some quick tests to find out what type of skin you have, as well as some tips on how to care for each skin type.

1 FIND YOUR BASIC SKIN TYPE

Dry skin, normal skin, or oily skin

Choose the answers that best describe your skin and add up the points to determine your skin type.

	YES	SOMEWHAT	NO
My face is greasy	3	2	1
My nose is shiny	3	2	1
My face is partially dry	1	2	3
My skin has a rough texture	3	2	1
I have acne	3	2	1
My skin feels moist	2	3	1
I have visible fine wrinkles	1	2	3
My skin looks dull	3	2	1
Makeup won't stay on	3	2	1
My skin is easily irritated	1	2	3

10–15 POINTS

Dry skin

Your skin produces little sweat and oil and is low on moisture. It's prone to roughness and fine wrinkles, so guard against dehydration and focus year-round on keeping it moisturized, regardless of the season. You'll see a difference in how your skin fares during the drier months.

16–20 POINTS

Normal skin

You have ideal skin with active metabolism. The downside is that it's sensitive to seasonal changes in the climate. Special care is needed during the transitional periods. Think "moisturize in summer" and "exfoliate in winter."

21–30 POINTS

Oily skin

Your skin produces a lot of oil, tending to acne and breakouts, and makeup comes off easily. Make a habit of exfoliating dead skin cells with facial scrub. But take care not to overwash your face. Also, hydrating your skin will help balance its moisture and oil content and regulate oil secretion.

PROBLEM TENDENCIES

Spring-summer skin and fall-winter skin

Check the items that apply. Your skin type is the one with more check marks.

SPRING-SUMMER SKIN

☐ I have visible pores on my forehead, nose, and chin
☐ Makeup won't stay on
☐ My skin tends to get shiny with oil
☐ I'm prone to acne and breakouts
☐ My skin has a rough texture
☐ I have deep lines around the eyes and mouth
☐ My T-zone is always oily
☐ My skin is oily but tends to peel
☐ I have irregular wrinkles
☐ My skin lacks clarity and freshness

FALL-WINTER SKIN

☐ My skin is tough and flaky
☐ Makeup doesn't sit well and blend with my skin
☐ I have fine lines around the eyes
☐ My skin is thin
☐ My complexion is fair
☐ My skin doesn't feel soft and moist
☐ My skin lacks elasticity
☐ My skin is rough around the chin
☐ My cheeks are purple-red
☐ My skin dries out toward the end of summer

Skincare for spring-summer skin

Spring-summer skin produces a lot of oil due to lack of moisture. Problems tend to occur in the spring and summer. People with this type of skin often wash their faces too often and are preoccupied with removing the oil. But overwashing your skin will only take away the needed moisture and induce excessive oil production. Make it your main mission to balance out your skin's moisture and oil content.

Spring mornings

1	Wash	Gel-type facial soap
2	Lotion	Brightening lotion
3	Serum	Vitamin C serum
4	Emulsion/cream	Emulsion with UV protection

Spring evenings

1	Cleanser	Milk-type cleanser
2	Lotion	Brightening lotion
3	Serum	Emulsion-type serum with vitamin A
4	Emulsion/cream	(Substitute with #3)

Summer mornings

1	Wash	Brightening facial soap
2	Lotion	Brightening lotion
3	Serum	Vitamin C serum
4	Emulsion/cream	Emulsion with UV protection

Summer evenings

1	Cleanser	Gel-type cleanser
2	Lotion	Brightening lotion
3	Serum	Vitamin C serum
4	Emulsion/cream	Brightening emulsion

Fall mornings

1 Wash	Gel-type facial soap
2 Lotion	Brightening lotion
3 Serum	Vitamin C serum
4 Emulsion/cream	Brightening emulsion or cream

Fall evenings

1 Cleanser	Mousse-type cleanser
2 Lotion	Astringent lotion
3 Serum	Moisturizing serum
4 Emulsion/cream	Moisturizing emulsion

Winter mornings

1 Wash	Mousse-type facial soap
2 Lotion	Astringent lotion
3 Serum	Moisturizing serum
4 Emulsion/cream	Moisturizing emulsion

Winter evenings

1 Cleanser	Cream-type cleanser
2 Lotion	Moisturizing lotion
3 Serum	Moisturizing serum
4 Emulsion/cream	Moisturizing cream

Skincare for fall-winter skin

Fall-winter skin is short on both moisture and oil. It tends to encounter problems with dryness, such as flaking and fine wrinkles, in the fall and winter months. But applying rich cream isn't the solution. First, you need to nurse the inner layers back to health, and then hydrate the surface. After charging the dermis with moisture and nutrients, seal your skin with cream to finish. Use moisturizing cream even during the summer.

Spring mornings

1	Wash	Mousse-type facial soap
2	Lotion	Moisturizing lotion
3	Serum	Moisturizing serum
4	Emulsion/cream	Moisturizing emulsion

Spring evenings

1	Cleanser	Emulsion-type cleanser
2	Lotion	Moisturizing lotion
3	Serum	Moisturizing serum
4	Emulsion/cream	Moisturizing emulsion or cream

Summer mornings

1	Wash	Gel-type facial soap
2	Lotion	Moisturizing brightening lotion
3	Serum	Moisturizing vitamin C serum
4	Emulsion/cream	Moisturizing emulsion or brightening cream

Summer evenings

1	Cleanser	Emulsion-type cleanser
2	Lotion	Moisturizing lotion
3	Serum	Moisturizing serum
4	Emulsion/cream	Moisturizing emulsion or cream

Fall mornings

1 Wash   Foam-type facial soap
2 Lotion   Moisturizing lotion
3 Serum   Anti-wrinkle serum
4 Emulsion/cream   Anti-wrinkle emulsion or cream

Fall evenings

1 Cleanser   Cream-type cleanser
2 Lotion   Moisturizing lotion
3 Serum   Moisturizing serum
4 Emulsion/cream   Anti-wrinkle, anti-dehydration lifting cream

Winter mornings

1 Wash   Mousse-type facial soap
2 Lotion   Moisturizing lotion
3 Serum   Lifting serum
4 Emulsion/cream   Moisturizing cream

Winter evenings

1 Cleanser   Cream-type cleanser
2 Lotion   Moisturizing lotion
3 Serum   Lifting serum
4 Emulsion/cream   Highly concentrated moisturizing cream

（英文版）美肌革命
The Japanese Skincare Revolution

2008 年 11 月 28 日　第 1 刷発行

著　者　佐伯 チズ
訳　者　横田 恵
撮　影　高山 浩数
編集協力　水井 真理子
発行者　富田 充
発行所　講談社インターナショナル株式会社
　　　　〒112-8652 東京都文京区音羽 1-17-14
　　　　電話　03-3944-6493（編集部）
　　　　　　　03-3944-6492（営業部・業務部）
　　　　ホームページ　www.kodansha-intl.com
印刷・製本所　大日本印刷株式会社